Raw Juicing

Raw Juicing

The Healthy, Easy and Delicious Way to Gain the Benefits of the Raw Food Lifestyle

Leslie Kenton
with Russell Cronin

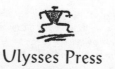

Ulysses Press

To all of those who seek the highs
but are devastated by the lows that usually follow
this little book is dedicated

❧

Published by: Ulysses Press
P.O. Box 3440
Berkeley, CA 94703
www.ulyssespress.com

ISBN-10: 1-56975-713-5
ISBN-13: 978-1-56975-713-0
Library of Congress Control Number: 2009902018

Printed in Canada by Transcontinental Printing

10 9 8 7 6 5 4 3 2 1

Acquisitions Editor: Nicholas Denton-Brown
Managing Editor: Claire Chun
Editor: Emma Silvers
Editorial and Production staff: Lauren Harrison, Kate Kellogg,
    Judith Metzener
Cover design: what!design @ whatweb.com
Cover photos: front, orange juice squeeze ©
istockphoto.com/redmonkey8; pomegranate © istockphoto.com/suzifoo;
pomegranate juice © istockphoto.com/gresei;
back © shutterstock.com/Elena Itsenko

Distributed by Publishers Group West

NOTE TO READERS
This book has been written and published strictly for informational purposes, and in no way should be used as a substitute for consultation with health-care professionals. You should not consider educational material herein to be the practice of medicine or to replace consultation with a physician or other medical practitioner. The author and publisher are providing you with information in this work so that you can have the knowledge and can choose, at your own risk, to act on that knowledge. The author and publisher also urge all readers to be aware of their health status and to consult health-care professionals before beginning any health program.

Contents

1

THE CHARGE

Hit the juice high. It will change your life. As soon as you begin to incorporate freshly extracted, raw vegetable and fruit juices into your lifestyle something amazing starts happening to you. First you will notice the terrific lift that just one glass of fresh juice can give you, particularly if taken first thing in the morning on an empty stomach. Ten to fifteen minutes after drinking it down, you feel yourself magically perking up. Your head clears and even your vision seems sharper; your abdomen tightens and your fingertips tingle. These are the characteristics of what we call the Raw Energy Rush, and we never tire of initiating people to the experience. Sometimes they're skeptical but are persuaded to try our freshly extracted juice because it tastes so delicious. Half an hour later they're back, with a gleam in their eye, demanding to know "what is the secret ingredient?"

Lifepower

Life is the secret—the most profound mystery of the universe—and raw juice is bursting with it. Raw juice is the most perfect fuel because it's easily assimilated to cleanse and nurture the body while supplying it with a full range of essential nutrients. That's all there is to it. Except, of course, that raw juice also has another property, a mysterious X factor, which scientists have yet to properly understand. It could be ascribed to the high redox potential of live juices or the inscrutable action of enzymes, but freshly extracted juices are bursting with a vital natural energy that is miraculous in its beneficial effect on the human body.

The nutritional and recuperative value of raw juice has been well known to doctors and natural health practitioners since the 19th century, when several of the most eminent pioneers in the field started experimenting with raw foods to improve their own health. The famous Rohsäft Kur (raw juice cure), developed by Dr. Max Bircher-Benner and Dr. Max Gerson in the early years of the 20th century, is acknowledged to be the single most potent short-term antidote to fatigue and stress, but until recently it's been the preserve of the privileged few who could afford to go to an exclusive health spa.

Now, with the advent of affordable domestic centrifugal juice extractors and high-tech nutrition research, the salvation of raw juice is within the reach of us all. Our raw juice cure, the Juice Blitz, can be undertaken over a weekend in the comfort of your own home, yet it is nothing less than life-changing—physically, mentally, and spiritually (see Chapter 4). Anybody who is sufficiently concerned about their own welfare to invest in a juicer can begin to experience the power of Raw Energy right away. Get into the routine of drinking raw juice on a regular basis and you will find that the more you drink of it, the better you'll feel.

Refresh Yourself

Replenishment is the immutable law of life. We require adequate supplies of air, food and water. Deprived of any one of these, we will expire in pretty short order. Water constitutes 70 percent of the human body and serves the crucial function within the body of transporting nutrients to its tissues and, in turn, removing waste products. If we failed to regularly replenish the water in our bodies which is lost through perspiration we would soon start to wilt. We all know what it's like to be dehydrated and to feel thirsty; a growing awareness of the need for plenty of clean water has spawned a huge industry selling bottled mineral water.

The soft drink industry is another rapidly growing business that churns out billions of dollars worth of glossy propaganda to persuade us that cans of carbonated syrup will satisfy our thirst and give us energy. There's even a breed of so-called sports drinks that claim not only to replace bodily fluids, but also to reinvigorate tired muscles. Actually, the last thing most of these synthetic products can offer your body is proper refreshment, and, while they may give you a sugar shock or a caffeine jolt, as a source of prolonged energy they are pretty useless.

So-called soft drinks bring nutritionally empty calories into your body which you can hardly afford. A 12-ounce can of soda contains, on average, seven teaspoons of sugar—about 40 grams. Sodas are full of chemicals to pollute your body and detour your liver's elimination processes. As for the "diet" varieties, aside from the proven fact that drinking them will do absolutely nothing to help you lose weight—

which presumably is why most women are attracted to them—they are an even more chemically unpleasant cocktail full of excess phosphorous and additives which only pollutes your body and further contributes to calcium loss from bones. Stay away from them. They are also full of phosphoric acid—the chemical used to etch glass—which, when your body tries to eliminate it via the kidneys, combines with calcium, leaching this vital mineral from bones, teeth, nails and hair. Sodas are major contributors to osteoporosis in women.

LIFEWATER

The kind of water your body craves and depends upon to function at peak efficiency does not come out of a tap, or from a bottle, but is only to be found in fresh fruits and vegetables. Your body can't make good use of the water in carbonated drinks, or beer, and so those fluids pass quickly through to the bladder. The water extracted from raw fruit and vegetables, however, has a unique, organic, living, quality. It is readily absorbed by the body. Because it is so rich in essential micronutrients, raw juice effectively replenishes lost energy. In fact, raw juice is the most profoundly refreshing thing you can drink.

The first reason you should abandon soft drinks and make raw juice your preferred beverage is because it tastes fantastic. If you've tried bottled carrot juice and didn't like it, don't be put off from tasting the real thing. Freshly extracted carrot juice is sweet, creamy and delicious. Mix it with apple juice and you have a whole drink that is perfectly balanced for your nutritional needs, and tastes so good that nobody in our experience has ever turned their nose up at it. Even children who are accustomed to saccharine-sweet carbonated drinks are amazed by just how good a glass of raw juice is, especially on a warm day. Some may complain that it's not ice-cold enough, but there's a good reason for that. To be most effective, raw juice is best drunk at room temperature. Ice dilutes your juice and makes it too cold to be quickly assimilated. If you love a "chill," keep your fresh produce in the fridge before juicing it.

Energize Your Life

Energy is the essence of life and the fundamental prerequisite for good health. A lack of steady, long-term energy is the precursor to disease. With energy, everything we seek from life becomes feasible and achievable. In both the plant and the animal kingdoms, the basic building block and source of energy is the cell, of which there are billions in your body. Cytology (the study of cells) reveals that these tiny powerhouses, in their almost infinite numbers, are what keep us energized and fully alive. Each type of cell not only performs its own specialized function but, when adequately supplied with oxygen, also produces the adenosine triphosphate (ATP) that fuels the body.

Endless Renewal

For our bodies to function at peak efficiency we must provide the optimum conditions for each cell to do its work. Cells require three things: oxygen, nutrients and the ability to expel their own waste. Given ideal conditions, as Dr. Alexis Carrel famously proved, they will live forever. He took some cells from the heart of a chicken and kept them in a nutrient bath which he changed every day in order to keep the cells detoxified. Chickens have a life expectancy of about seven years, but these chicken cells were kept alive for 32 years. In fact, they outlived Carrel himself and only died because one day the lab assistant forgot to renew their nutrient bath.

In order to be fit and healthy and to live a long and active life, we need plenty of fresh air and the vital nourishment that comes from eating whole foods. It may seem obvious to us now, but it's only in comparatively recent times that mankind has come to the gradual realization that the condition of the human body is inextricably bound up with the quality of the food we ingest and the air we breathe. Over the past 100 years, the quality of both our food and air—and, consequently, our ability to be healthy—have declined quite dramatically. Because we now live in an environment that is increasingly toxic, we need the most effective form of nutrition we can get in order to combat its degenerative, aging effects and to revitalize our bodies. That's where live juices come in.

Rah Rah Raw!

Fresh fruit and vegetables are the best possible foods. In their raw natural state, they contain the most valuable range of nutrients that the human body needs, in the perfect synergy and in the form they can be most easily utilized. Because of their high water content, they are readily digestible and tend to cleanse and nurture body, mind and spirit. Fresh fruit and vegetables also have another quality which is intangible and cannot be quantified, but could be compared to an electrical charge. We call it Raw Energy, and the most immediate way to experience its power is by drinking raw juice.

All our energy is ultimately derived from the food we eat, but the body has to expend energy in order to break down and digest our food before we can derive any nutritional benefit from it. Without proper digestion there can be no such thing as good nutrition. By extracting the juices of fruits and vegetables, removing the fiber, you can provide the body with an excellent source of nutrition that is virtually predigested, so that it is absorbed into the body with the minimum expenditure of energy. In fact, freshly extracted, nutrient-rich live juice is nothing but liquid Raw Energy.

We are not all that fond of cars, but just for a moment think of your body as a motor car. Do you want to drive around in some old crock that guzzles fuel and belches black fumes, or would you prefer a faster, cleaner and sleeker machine? You would probably rather have a smart car, just as you'd rather have a healthy body. Think of juicing as a way of supercharging your engine with fuel injection in order to maximize its performance.

Poor Elvis

Consider Elvis Presley. The quintessential icon of rock 'n' roll, the King is one of the most crucial figures of the 20th century. But his life ended prematurely and in tragedy. The young Elvis had it all: the voice, the looks and the sex appeal. But he also had a fatal flaw. Brought up dirt poor and unable to afford to eat well as a youngster should, he developed a fetish for rich and fatty foods, of which he consumed more and more as he got older. This compulsive eating of junk foods made Elvis neither happy nor healthy, so he started taking all sorts of drugs to feel better. But that didn't help, it just made him into an addict and his diet got steadily worse, making him increasingly sluggish and miserable.

There is still some debate about exactly *what* killed Elvis. Was it the lethal cocktail of drugs washing around inside him? Or was it an old-fashioned heart attack brought about by his dismal diet? Everyone knows *how* Elvis died, however. The King was on his throne when he had his fatal seizure, straining to force a bowel movement. According to the coroner's report, there were pounds of impacted feces in his bowels when he fell off the toilet seat, and his vital spark was extinguished.

The undignified death of Elvis Presley serves as a dire warning to us all. How could a man so fabulously rich, both in terms of talent and material wealth, live so appallingly and die in such sordid circumstances? If only someone had explained to Elvis the guiding principles of a decent diet, persuaded him to cut down on his intake of cheeseburgers and convinced him that the way to control his weight was not with crash diets and amphetamine pills, but by eating right, not only would he have felt better able to take charge of his career (he might have stuck to singing and spared us the films), Elvis the Pelvis might still be around to entertain us.

Take Out the Garbage

What nobody taught Elvis is the simple fact that everything you put into your body must be either assimilated or eliminated. Assimilation is the process of extracting from your food the nutrients that your body needs; elimination is the process of excreting the residues that your body can't use. Elvis Presley lived almost exclusively on indigestible junk food that clogged his colon with putrefying waste and made him chronically constipated. Because he was unable to eliminate the toxic waste of the nutritionally worthless foods he was eating, the garbage built up in his body to the point where it killed him.

It's true enough that we are what we eat, but it's more accurate to say that we are what we assimilate. No less important than efficient assimilation is the prompt elimination of food wastes that will otherwise accumulate in the colon and decay, breeding putrefactive bacteria that release toxins that get into the bloodstream, spreading all sorts of sickness throughout the body. More and more people are discovering that to stay healthy, therefore, it's vitally important to keep your colon clean and to give your body a chance to process the food you put into it. This is why the practice of colonic irrigation has become so fashionable.

Elvis is an extreme example, but the majority of people living in the developed world, where it's practically impossible to easily avoid eating any processed food, suffer from constipation to some degree. Even if you're accustomed to an effortless bowel movement on a daily basis, you may still be constipated. That may seem like an alarming statement, and, to demonstrate the truth of it, we're going to have to ask you to do something that you may find distasteful: take a good look at your stools. (This is not so hard if you happen to live in one of the European countries where the use of raw juice was pioneered. Germans and Swiss appear to be a lot less squeamish about the consistency of their stools: their lavatories have a platform where they can be examined before flushing.)

CLEAN SWEEP

Before taking a look at your feces, let's take a moment to consider the process by which feces is produced. Food passes through the body, from the esophagus via the stomach and gastrointestinal tract, where it's broken down and nutrients are assimilated into the body. The residues of digested food pass from the small intestine into the colon in liquid form and are moved along by the action of peristalsis to be eliminated from the bowels. When the food we eat is raw and unprocessed, the fibers it contains act as kind of intestinal broom, assisting peristaltic activity and promoting efficient elimination. When food is denatured by processing, however, the action is more like a filthy mop that leaves a trail of slime coating the intestinal walls and making the colon sluggish and slow. The longer food waste lies around in the colon, the more moisture is extracted from it and the harder and more compacted it becomes.

The literal meaning of "constipation" is to press together. Constipated feces is closely compacted and comes out looking like fat cigars that have been extruded from the colon, which is exactly what happens when one has to strain to force a bowel movement. Feces excreted from a healthy colon is much more mushy and fluffy around the edges; it passes smoothly from the body and breaks up easily when the toilet is flushed. Without wanting to be facetious, you know you're working well when you produce little fluffy stools.

We've talked about how raw juice contains all sorts of vital nutrients and how its high water content ensures rapid assimilation, exerting minimum strain on the digestive system. There is nothing in raw juice that your body cannot use and, therefore, nothing that it need work to expel. Instead, the body can concentrate on getting rid of old waste. The action of raw juice will encourage that by irrigating the intestine and causing a chain reaction in the colon that can have explosive results! This gentle laxative effect, which is particularly pronounced with fruit juices, is highly beneficial because it helps the body to detoxify itself, restoring its chemical balance and to providing the ideal environment for biological regeneration.

Rejuvenate Your Body

As you become accustomed to juicing, and to the effect of raw juice on your bowel movements, you may well shed excess weight. As your colon cleanses itself and your metabolism becomes more efficient, and so long as you are not continually clogging your system with junk foods, the body will lose excess fat and revert to it's natural weight. You start to feel fitter and younger than you have in years, and you get used to old friends telling you how well you look. What's more, when you see yourself in the mirror, you even *look* younger; your complexion seems smoother and wrinkles recede.

This is no illusion. Raw juice really is a veritable elixir of life. The energy it contains has the potential to rejuvenate your body in a way that quite literally makes you younger. What makes us old is not merely the passing years but environmental poisons, inadequate food and the mental stresses that living in such an undernourished state inevitably cause. These factors cause an acidic chemical imbalance within the body that is redressed by raw juice, which tends to alkalinize the system. By restoring this harmonious balance, the juice provides the ideal environment for the body to repair cellular damage and to rebuild itself from within.

Perhaps the biggest factor in premature aging is the free radical particles in atmospheric pollution, which we will be discussing in the next chapter. These biochemical bullies vandalize our bodies at a cellular level, and the best way to combat them is to drink raw juice. The natural antioxidants and enzymes within raw juice are not only capable of arresting the process of premature aging, they work together to actually reverse it. There are even well-documented case histories of people who've found that a regular intake of raw juice has caused their gray hair to revert to its original color. Who says you can't turn the clock back?

Expand Your Mind

Never forget that body and the mind are inseparable, interdependent, synergistic parts of the same whole—you. People working in the soul-sapping environment of, say, a modern office building will reach for coffee and carbonated drinks in the middle of the afternoon in the hope that these will give them enough mental energy to make it through to the end of another hectic day. Then they experience a corresponding energy slump on the way home, arriving irritable and exhausted and good for nothing but going early to bed. The end result of living like this is a kind of chronic fatigue that often manifests itself as indifferent, fatalistic lethargy.

As you master the basic principles of juicing and get into the practice of drinking raw juice on a daily basis, energizing your life and rejuvenating your body, you will find yourself becoming better able to cope with the debilitating stresses of modern life. Raw juice will help you to build the stamina to cope, and it will also transform the way you see the world around you. As your body rebalances itself, you'll find that your moods will stabilize, too. Trivialities will cease to upset you and you will be able to keep things in perspective. Detoxifying the system and flushing your colon with raw juice actually helps you to think more clearly and rationally, concentrate for longer and maintain a more optimistic frame of mind. This is the state we call Juice High, and, unlike the high you get from coffee or drugs, it is perfectly possible to stay high on raw juice all of the time.

Drinking raw juice is not like doing drugs. Drug users often say they are seeking enlightenment, to "expand their minds," but by artificially altering their perceptions with chemicals, they may be doing themselves damage. Whether or not drugs do long-term harm, their effects are temporary and usually followed by a "crash" when the drug wears off. (Drinking raw juice, by the way, is the best possible thing you can do to recover from the after-effects of drug abuse or excessive drinking.) People take drugs to get "out their heads," but raw juice will have the opposite effect, making you feel high yet at the same time more "normal," well centered, standing straight with both feet on the ground and better able to cope with the bows and arrows of outrageous reality. In short, live juices can help you have your cake and eat it too.

Best of all, an abundance of raw energy makes you feel fully alive and properly connected to the world around you. This world can seem such a tiresome and threatening place that sometimes you wonder how you can keep going, but thanks to the power of raw energy you can rise above it, learn to live with fresh zest and have more fun than you may have thought possible.

Free Your Spirit

Imagine how much more confident you would feel if you could stop worrying about the way you look in the eyes of other people. Living with the power of raw energy enables you to stop fretting about possible pimples or blemishes because you will know that your complexion is clear and radiantly healthy. Think what life might be like if, instead of trying to kick-start yourself with strong coffee in the mornings, you could drink a glass of raw juice and almost immediately feel refreshed, alert and eager to see what another day has in store. This is the liberating effect of the Juice High.

The eyes are the windows of the soul, and, if you look into the eyes of a person who has been juicing for a while, you'll notice something extraordinary there. For sure, those pellucid pools are almost transparently clear and literally shining with health, but there's another, indefinable quality in that level gaze. It might be called serenity. People who are in control of their health are in control of their destiny, able to work harder and more effectively to fulfill their wildest dreams. We believe you can't get higher than that.

2

GET SET!

At the beginning of the 21st century, it's becoming increasingly obvious that something has gone terribly wrong with the way that we live on this planet. In a little over a hundred years, since the start of the Industrial Revolution, mankind has squandered and come close to using up most of Mother Nature's once bountiful resources. Meanwhile, man has so befouled the soil, air and water upon which we depend for life that scarcely anywhere on Earth remains untainted by pollution. It can hardly be a coincidence that the inexorable degradation of our environment has been steadily matched by the gradual biological degeneration of our bodies and our spirits.

We live in an environment that is increasingly toxic. At the same time, the quality of our food has been compromised, so that it is often inadequate to provide us with enough proper nutrition to be able to withstand disease. However, there is something you can do to protect yourself, to boost your immune system and promote optimum health. That is simply to get a juicer and start to consume freshly extracted raw fruit and vegetable juices on a daily basis.

Food Glut

Of all the changes that technology has wrought, none is more profound and potentially catastrophic than the revolution that's taken place in our eating habits over the past century. Commercial considerations, rather than concern for human health, have been allowed to dictate the way in which our food is produced, processed and distributed. Crops are grown in chemically fertilized soils, doused with pesticides and then made into products that are packaged to be shipped over long distances and stored for extended periods. All these complicated modern practices conspire to destroy the wholesome quality of the foodstuffs we can most easily afford to buy from the local supermarket. The convenience foods that dominate the diets of most of us privileged enough to be living in the affluent, developed world have had their nutritional integrity destroyed and their natural goodness systematically stripped from them and replaced with a range of artificial additives to enhance their taste and texture and to prolong their shelf lives as long as possible.

The consequences of living on a diet composed largely of the kind of highly processed foodstuffs that fill most shopping carts are easy to see when you walk down the street. Just look how many hyperactive, phlegmatic or fat people there are! Refined foods are loaded with excessive amounts of fats and sugars but offer the body practically nothing in terms of nutrition, failing to adequately satisfy our appetite for real food and tempting us to compulsively overeat.

FAT CHANCE

Widespread obesity is a relatively new phenomenon. It is also a contributing factor in a range of chronic degenerative diseases that have become the biggest killers of modern times, such as heart disease and cancer. Although it is perfectly possible to subsist on a diet of microwave-ready meals, it's not possible to thrive. For such a diet is deficient in many of the essential nutrients that are abundantly available in fresh fruits and vegetables. Common sense tells you that, unless you get your quota of vitamins, you quickly start to feel run down and become susceptible to any stray virus that's going around.

A poor diet undermines good health and leaves you in poor shape to cope with the stresses and strains of modern life but, much worse, it's bad for the soul. The physiological effect of a high-gunk diet—that's one that tends to clog your system with garbage that's nutritionally worthless and hard to digest—is to slow you down, making you feel heavy and, ultimately, depressed. But don't get too down on yourself about your eating habits. It's easy enough to get juicing and start doing something positive about it.

Nix on Smog

The internal combustion engine has proven to be the most destructive invention of the 20th century, and it's going to be difficult to explain to future generations why we allowed their air to be poisoned by exhaust fumes and condemned them to grow up with a range of respiratory illnesses caused by pollution. Those of us who are lucky enough to live in rural areas are largely dependent on our cars, and, out in the country, it's possible to persuade ourselves that the impact of the motor car has been limited to the main arterial routes and the bypasses that protect our town centers from heavy traffic. But in urban areas it's impossible to escape the oppressive pollution spewed out by cars.

Breathe in by the side of the road and savor the acrid cocktail of sulphur dioxide and carbon monoxide, liberally laced with benzene and hydrocarbons. The air quality in our cities is so poor that cyclists customarily wear masks to filter out the most poisonous particles. Sometimes, especially in the summer, when the ozone gets totally out of control, it gets so bad that people with respiratory problems are officially advised to stay indoors. And we just carry on coping as this crazy state of affairs gets steadily worse.

BIOCHEMICAL CHAOS

Your body is a biochemical battleground in which the bad guys are the free radicals, which are particularly prevalent in car exhaust fumes. Scientifically, free rads are molecules with an unpaired electron, which makes them highly reactive and inclined to stabilize themselves by attracting another electron from any other molecule, particularly the lipids in cell membranes. Cells are the fundamental building blocks of our bodily tissues, and, by knocking out a few of these blocks in a process called "lipid peroxidation," free radicals can bring the whole lot tumbling down by causing an ever-amplifying series of chain reactions that leads to the destruction of tissues. That's the way smoking and breathing heavily polluted air corrodes our vitality, causes cancer and makes us old before our time.

Still, what can you do? Walking around in a hi-tech gas mask is hardly practical, so you'd better ensure you get yourself a plentiful supply of the fresh vitamins that can prevent or retard free radical damage. You need plenty of A, C and E, the so-called antioxidant vitamins, as well as zinc, selenium, the sulphur-containing amino acids such as methionine, and other recently discovered plant based antioxidant compounds which are found only in fresh fruits and vegetables, to protect yourself against the degenerative effects of pollution. The best way to ensure an adequate supply is to drink plenty of freshly extracted raw juice.

Don't Wilt

Before World War II, all crops were grown without the use of chemicals, which is to say organically. The organic matter in healthy soil is a hotbed of biological activity that creates fertility and promotes the growth of strong, healthy plants. Artificial chemicals interfere with that vital process, stripping the soil of its natural goodness and depriving the plants gown in it of the essential minerals and other microsubstances they need to thrive.

A 12-year study of vegetables grown with composted manure compared to those grown with artificial fertilizers showed marked discrepancies in the levels of vitamins, amino acids, iron, potassium, calcium and phosphorous. Destroy the soil's organic matter through chemical farming and slowly, but inexorably, the health of the people and animals that live on the foods grown in it will be undermined and their resistance to disease will be compromised.

The body has an amazing ability to compensate for missing nutrients, but after years of eating nutritionally depleted foods, widespread deficiencies are becoming apparent and all sorts of metabolic distortions follow. Being fat is the most obvious one, but perhaps the most insidious effect of the modern diet is the imbalance of sodium and potassium that develops in many peoples' bodies.

Sodium and potassium are nutritional antagonists that act synergistically in the body to regulate the osmotic pressure on the walls of each cell. When properly balanced, theses two minerals also transmit electrochemical impulses throughout the body, keeping the whole organism vibrant. Too much sodium or too little potassium and the organism starts to wilt, causing the kind of chronic fatigue that has you reaching for chocolate or coffee just to keep going. That is what's happening to masses of people nowadays who have too much salt in their diet, promoting acidity in the body and undermining its resilience. What they need is potassium and the best way to get it—you guessed it—is by drinking raw juice.

Contaminated Carrots

The humble carrot is king of the vegetables, and it's the most versatile veggie when it comes to juicing. Its glorious orange color comes from beta carotene, which the body converts to vitamin A, and carrots also contain the other crucial antioxidants, vitamins C and E, as well as B, D, G and K and the minerals calcium, sodium, potassium, iron and phosphorus. Carrot juice is composed of a combination of elements that nourish the entire system, helping the body to normalize its weight and restore its chemical balance. CJ is incredibly good for you, but recent reports have suggested that eating carrots could be harmful because they contain poisonous pesticide residues.

Not long ago, the U.K.'s Pesticides Safety Directorate issued a warning after scientists found pesticide residues in carrots 25 times higher than they had expected and, in some cases, three times higher than the accepted safety level. The Food Minister was moved to advise the public to remove the tops and peel all carrots, as if that would make them safe. Sadly, the systemic organophosphates concerned don't stop at the skin, they penetrate the whole vegetable. It is disgraceful that the nutritional integrity of the noble carrot should have been debased in this way, but the possible presence of pesticide residues doesn't mean we shouldn't drink carrot juice. Naturally, it is always preferable to use organic produce wherever possible. This will give you a far better balance of vitamins and minerals. But thankfully it is the fibers of vegetables that tend to collect most of the injurious toxins. So if you can't go organic you can still benefit. By removing the fiber and extracting the juice, we're able to enjoy the goodness of carrots and minimize the effects of the poisons that have entered our food chain.

Degenerative Health

Modern medicine has more or less eradicated the diseases that used to regularly decimate the population, and people these days live longer than ever, but do we live better? In fact, statistics demonstrate that we're not getting any healthier. We are becoming increasingly prone to chronic degenerative diseases that are the result of inadequate nutrition. The health of any organism is directly dependent on the quality of the nutrients it receives and human beings require a massively complex variety of vitamins, minerals and amino acids.

Not only do our bodies need the full range of nutrients to be healthy, but they also need them to be available in the form in which they can most readily be assimilated and used. That means in the raw. Raw fruits and vegetables have uniquely healthful properties that science has yet to fully comprehend. Since scientists cannot formulate into pills nutrients they haven't yet discovered, the biggest synthetic vitamin pill you can buy can never compensate for a lack of the natural goodness that is only contained within raw fruits and vegetables.

Good health should not be defined as the absence of disease, but as a vital, dynamic condition in which we feel positively charged and fully able to take whatever life has to throw at us. In order to attain and maintain that blissful state, it's vitally important that we consume adequate quantities of fresh food, and the easiest way to ensure that you get all the vitamins you need is to drink raw juices.

Enzymes Work

The simple reason why raw juices are so great for you is because they deliver the most complete range of nutrients in their most vital form, straight into your system suspended in water from an organic source and brimming with enzymes. That's why we think of it as Raw Energy. Enzymes are the intangible living elements that act as the catalyst for innumerable chemical reactions within the body, promoting efficient assimilation and enabling the metabolic processes that support high levels of energy and promote good health.

You might derive the same benefit from eating two pounds of raw carrots, for instance, as from drinking a glass of carrot juice, but not nearly so efficiently. The insoluble fibers in root vegetables cannot be digested and are expelled from the body via the colon, where it acts as an intestinal broom, sweeping out bacterial debris and promoting efficient elimination. That's why the Total Juices that we will come to later can be so good. They make a wonderful companion to the lighter juices from which the fiber has been removed. The two kinds of juices are also delicious mixed together to make one drink. A decent amount of fiber in the diet is essential for a good health, but the process of breaking it down takes time and energy.

The removal of the fibers in the extraction of raw juices enables the juice to be assimilated immediately, sometimes in a matter of minutes, without exerting the digestive system. Because it is mostly water, the juice tends to cleanse and to nurture the system while supplying all the cells and tissues of the body with the vital nutrients and nutritional enzymes they need.

Get Smart

There's nothing controversial in the suggestion that eating fresh fruit and vegetables will significantly reduce your chances of dying prematurely from heart disease or cancer. The World Health Organization recommends that we eat at least a pound of fresh fruit and vegetables every day. A group of government-sponsored programs called 5 A Day is backing an initiative to encourage people to consume a minimum of five portions of fruit and vegetables per day. The average American eats one and one-half servings of vegetables and one serving of fruit per day, and many avoid fruit and vegetables altogether. It's hardly surprising, then, that heart disease is the leading cause of death in the United States.

It's not just adults who require the Raw Energy of fresh foods to thrive. Unborn babies are particularly vulnerable, and thousands have been born with spina bifida because their mothers were deficient in folic acid during the first six weeks of pregnancy, perhaps before many of them even realized they were pregnant. Folic acid is a soluble vitamin, a member of the B complex, which assists the formation of DNA. It's abundant in green vegetables like broccoli but is easily destroyed by cooking.

How often were we told while growing up to eat up our greens or we wouldn't be big and strong? Many children refuse to eat enough fresh vegetables because they say they don't like the taste. Sadly, many kids these days are addicted to sugar and so used to sloppy convenience foods that they can't be bothered to chew whole foods properly. But fresh juices are easy to drink and it's no problem to persuade children to take them since they taste delicious.

Get Juiced

It's not just children who instinctively know what's good for them. We all have the capability to listen to what our bodies are telling us and to act accordingly by feeding ourselves the vital nutrition we subconsciously crave. The body and mind are not separate entities, but are completely interdependent so that the foods we consume dictate not only our physical well-being, but our moods and ability to think clearly. When the system gets clogged, the signals get confused so that, after years on a junk diet, we get out of touch with our bodies.

As soon as you start to incorporate freshly extracted raw fruits and vegetable juices into your lifestyle you will begin to slow the build-up of toxins in your body, and, as you continue to take raw juices on a regular basis, the deadly degenerative effects of a junk diet will be reversed. This process of detoxification may be gradual or it may be quite dramatic, depending on the enthusiasm with which you take to juicing, but its effects are always remarkable.

Any raw juice is better than none at all, but if you use your juice well and take it on a daily basis you will begin to notice a subtle transformation in the way you think and approach the world around you. Once you've mastered the basic principles of juicing that are outlined in the next chapter and started yourself on a program of detoxification and regeneration using the power of raw juice, as discussed in Chapters Four and Chapter Five, the process of transformation will be virtually complete. You may find yourself thinking more profound thoughts or better able to concentrate for longer periods of time. Or you might just come to the realization that since you started juicing, not only has your health perked up, you feel positively happy.

3

GET JUICED

Harmony is the underlying principle of life, the universe and everything. Without harmony there is discord and chaos. In Chapter One we talked about how the human body is constantly striving to cleanse itself and to restore internal harmony. In Chapter Two, we discussed the way in which environmental pollution and inadequate nutrition interfere with the way the human body works, compromising its ability to withstand infection and making us ill. All illnesses can be regarded as manifestations of disharmony within the human body.

The internal environment of the body requires perfect harmony for all the metabolic processes that animate your body and enable you to live a fully active and healthy life to work properly. Breathing polluted air and eating processed foods replete with sugar, junk fats and refined carbohydrates (not to mention bad habits like drinking and smoking) conspire to create excess acidity and a chemical imbalance within the body. All raw juices have a strongly alkalinizing effect, tipping the pH balance back to normal, helping to restore harmony and enabling the body to cleanse and heal itself.

Juice It

There are three clearly defined stages in the body's utilization of food: appropriation (eating and digestion), assimilation (taking in nutrients) and elimination (expelling waste products). While all these activities are always taking place to some extent, the function of each is heightened at different times during the course of a day. If you've ever slumped on the sofa after a big meal, unable to move, you'll know how much energy the process of breaking down food in the stomach requires. If you really stuff yourself, your body is forced to close down some of your other physiological functions while it comes to grips with digesting.

Because it requires so much energy, the body prefers to do most of the hard work of assimilation at night, while you sleep. By the time you wake up in the morning, you will have moved into the elimination cycle. This is not a matter of having a single bowel movement before breakfast, but a deep and thorough cleansing at the cellular level, with wastes being expelled via all the organs of elimination, including the skin and lungs, as well as the bowels and urinary tract. The elimination cycle lasts throughout the morning, and that is the best time to take raw juices, particularly those freshly extracted from fruit.

Fruit juices are great for getting you moving in the mornings. All fruit contains fructose, the natural sugar that your body can use for fuel, and is usually around 90 percent water, promoting prompt elimination. When perfectly ripe, fruit also contains its own digestive enzymes and is therefore virtually predigested—it passes rapidly through the stomach and into the intestines. Of course, fruit juices can cause a rapid rise in blood sugar, so diabetics and people who are prone to yeast infections should be careful how they use them, but most people will find the effect of a glass of raw fruit juice for breakfast quite invigorating. Drink a glass of freshly extracted watermelon or pineapple or pink grapefruit juice on an empty stomach, and within 15 minutes you'll be wide awake and ready to rock.

It is always best to take fruits or their juices on an empty stomach, since they cannot be as effective if their passage through the stomach is impeded by undigested food. In fact, resolving to consume nothing but raw juices and fruit from the moment you get up until lunchtime could well be the healthiest lifestyle decision you ever make. As the day progresses, incorporate more and more vegetables into your juices and switch their emphasis from sweet to savory.

Get Freshness

Freshness is the first principle of good juicing. When buying fresh produce, don't let yourself be sold on overripe fruit that's started to "turn" or soft and sad-looking vegetables with limp leaves. Choose only the most perfectly ripe fruits and vegetables, and don't buy more than you can use over a couple of days. You will be going through a lot of produce, but don't be tempted to buy in bulk unless you're sure you're going to use it up. While it's often not necessary to peel the produce you'll be juicing, it's essential to wash it thoroughly under cold running water, using a scrubbing brush if necessary.

Freshly extracted juices must be drunk as soon as they are made, before their raw energy expires. The nutrients in raw juice are highly volatile and will begin to deteriorate as soon as they are in contact with fresh air, so that the juice's essential vitality is quickly lost. If you want to demonstrate this for yourself, leave a glass of raw juice to stand for just a few minutes, and you'll see how quickly it separates into a clear liquid (water) with a scummy head on top. It's a lot less inviting than the vividly colored fluid you started with. Stir the scum back into the liquid before drinking it, and you'll notice a marked deterioration in the taste.

It's best not to try storing raw juices, but they can be kept in the fridge for a couple of hours, with a lid on the container. When going on a trip, or forced to spend the day in the alien environment of an office, we do find it beneficial to take along a container of raw juice to keep us going. Use a large, wide-necked, insulated thermos and pack it with ice cubes before pouring in your freshly extracted juice. That way the juice will keep for half a day or longer without losing too much of its wholesomeness, and it will certainly offer superior refreshment to canned soft drinks.

The Basics

So far, we've talked about fresh fruits and vegetables in more or less the same breath, but before you begin juicing it's important to understand that the two types of juice act within the body in quite different ways. Basically, fruit is liquid brain fuel that is particularly useful for detoxifying your body and clearing you mind, while vegetables provide the nutritional blocks for rebuilding the metabolic machinery of your body.

Some juice enthusiasts will warn you not to combine fruit and vegetable juices in the same glass, lest they give you gas and cause embarrassing flatulence. While this can happen, it is certainly not an absolute rule. The two types of juice can be combined satisfactorily, but in general they don't tend to taste so good together. The exceptions are carrot and apple, which can be mixed with anything.

CARROT IS KING

During the last world war, propagandists covered up the invention of radar by trying to persuade the enemy that allied fighter pilots were eating so many carrots that they could see in the dark! This hyperbole does, however, contain a grain of truth. Carrots have been repeatedly shown to nourish the optic nerve and significantly improve eyesight in general and night vision in particular. This is but one of the healing properties of the humble carrot, which is a rich source of beta carotene, the vegetable pigment that gives them their glorious orange color and which the body converts into the cancer-fighting antioxidant vitamin A.

It's hard to overemphasize the healthful properties of carrots, which contain an abundance of vitamins and a combination of nutrients which nourish the entire system, helping to normalize weight and restore chemical balance. When it comes to juicing, the carrot is king. It is the most versatile vegetable with the sweetest juice. If you've only ever tried bottled carrot juice and didn't like it, don't be put off from trying freshly extracted CJ, which tastes sublime.

CJ—COOL JUICE

The carotene content of carrots varies considerably and is reflected in the color. Carrots bought from the supermarket are sometimes almost fluorescent, while organic carrots are a much deeper shade of orange, indicating a much higher concentration of carotene. When buying carrots, choose those with the darkest color. Although size doesn't really matter, many of the recipes in this book refer to "medium-sized" carrots, around six inches in length.

Whichever variety you use, you'll need about a pound of carrots to make ten fluid ounces. As a rule of thumb, we think that half a dozen medium carrots will yield about half a pint of juice. Scrub them under cold running water and remove the tops and ends, but it is not necessary to peel carrots before putting them through the juicer.

Carrot & Apple

Carrot and apple—don't call it Crapple—is the most basic juice cocktail and it tastes so good that, in our experience, nobody has ever turned their nose up at it! Use the *whole* apple except for the woody stem. Apple seeds contain important nourishment, too. Start by combining equal parts of the two juices and experiment until you find the proportions that suit you—half and half perhaps, or one part apple to two parts carrot (see page 176).

Carrot & Orange

A classic breakfast juice and lots of peoples' favorite, carrot and orange is especially rich in vitamin C and good for guarding against colds. Simply peel the rind from an orange, but leave the pith, and put the whole fruit through the juicer together with four carrots (see page 176).

Carrot Milk

You can enhance the natural creaminess of freshly extracted carrot juice by adding soymilk, which contains plenty of protein and won't clog the body like cow's milk does. If you're feeling adventurous and enjoy parsnips (which have been called "anemic carrots"), try adding the juice of a single small parsnip root—scrubbed, topped and tailed, but not peeled—to three or four carrots. Then top up the glass with about ¾ cup soymilk. A little grated nutmeg adds another intriguing dimension to the flavor (see page 177).

Carrot, Beet, Celery & Tomato

This is a great recipe to experiment with when you are beginning to explore the earthiness of beet and all its blessings (see page 177).

APPLES ARE AMAZING!

If an apple a day keeps the doctor away, a glass or two of freshly extracted apple juice will keep you regular, boost your immunity to colds and keep your hair and nails looking lustrous. Apples are full of the soluble dietary fiber pectin, which makes the juice cloudy, gives it a delightfully creamy texture and cleans out toxins and relieves constipation in the body. Apples are also rich in beta carotene and vitamin C, as well as several B-complex vitamins, including B6, and the mineral potassium.

Like the carrot is the most versatile vegetable when it comes to juicing, apples are the most useful fruit. Apple juice can happily be mixed with any vegetable juice. As such, it is particularly useful in enabling those who are new to juicing to slowly acclimatize themselves to the earthy, wild, raw taste of some freshly extracted juices.

Start off by incorporating a lot of apple and gradually reduce the proportion as you become accustomed to the taste and texture of raw juice.

You may be familiar with the taste of juice pressed from various varieties of apple, but you might be surprised by how sweetly smooth and creamy freshly extracted apple juice is. There are dozens of apple varieties, each with its own distinct flavor, and it's fun to try each one as it crops up. In general, you'll find that the greener the apple, the sharper its juice. Golden Delicious are popular, but we find Pippins ideal.

There's no need to peel apples (in fact it's better if you don't) but do wash them thoroughly. Remove the stalk, but not the core. Simply chop them in half and put them through the juicer.

Apple & Pear

Apples and pears are closely related, but pear trees are less hardy and the fruit more perishable. Pear juice is thick, mild and versatile. It mixes well with other juices, and can be a useful substitute for apple in many recipes. Pears should be washed and the stem removed, then cut to fit your juicer. Mix the juice of two pears with the juice of two apples and drink it down promptly, since this combination oxidizes quickly (see page 174).

Apple, Pear & Berries

Berries are intensely flavored vitamin bombs that tend to be high in potassium and contain a remarkable range of other trace elements. Berries have been shown to be particularly good for fighting the flu and preventing cancer. Strawberries, raspberries, blackberries...in fact any berry works well when blended with apple juice, or apple and pear. Juice two apples, one pear and as many berries as you like or can fit into the glass (see page 174).

By the way, berries are replete with something called ellagic acid—a natural plant phenol that is believed to be a powerful anticancer/antiaging compound. Researchers working with it believe that ellagic acid probably has protective properties because it is taken up by receptor sites that are also used by chemically induced carcinogens. Animal experiments have demonstrated just how powerful a protective effect ellagic acid-containing foods have when researchers fed mice on them and then deliberately applied a nasty cancer-causing polycyclic aromatic hydrocarbon (PAH) to the skin for several weeks. The berry eaters had 45 percent fewer tumors than the control group, and the latency period before they appeared was stretched from six to ten weeks. Berries are also high in potassium and rich in iron. Some, like black currants and red currants, also contain GLA, while others, like cranberries, are great for clearing urinary tract and bladder infections.

Apple Zinger
This is a terrific breakfast-time enlivener that perks up the whole system and really wakes up your taste buds (see page 174).

TAKING THE PITH
When juicing citrus fruit, remove the peel, but leave as much of the white pith as you like to get the full benefit of the bioflavonoids contained within it, which help the body to absorb vitamin C. Bioflavonoids are powerful plant-based antioxidants. They also have an ability to strengthen the capillaries in the body, which carry nutrients to the cells via the blood stream. This means better circulation

and smoother, more beautiful skin. The juice of citrus fruits squeezed on a conventional cone-shaped juicer often has bits of pith floating in it, which have an unpleasant feel in the mouth, it also tends to taste sharp and to cause acidity within the body. Juice that's made using a centrifugal extractor, however, is a whole food in which the citric acid is neutralized by the bioflavonoids, providing the body with a well-balanced drink that can be readily assimilated. It's also absolutely delicious and has a wonderful creamy texture that is quite unlike squeezed juice.

Citrus juices are jam-packed with fruit sugar and bursting with vitamin C, helping to crank up the immune system and providing instant energy. We find a big glass of frothy pink grapefruit juice just the thing to get us started on a miserable, wet winter morning.

THE WHOLE JUICE

The seeds in fruits can be important sources of nutrients as well. For instance, orange and apple seeds are enormously rich in nutrients that are found in the fruit. The orange seed, for example, has nine times more calcium, seven times more magnesium and more potassium than an equal amount of orange juice. Apple seeds have five times more potassium than extracted apple juice. There is some evidence that certain seeds—those from the rose family such as cherries, peaches, plums, apricots and apples—contain a very small amount of a chemical called amygdaline, which is believed to release minute quantities of cyanide. However, this is not anything that one should be overly concerned about since you would have to consume 50 to 100 apricot pits to take in a harmful dose. We do not suggest you put apricot pits into the juicer, but apple and orange seeds are fine.

GO WITH THE FLOW

Raw juices are incredibly rich in nutrients and they have a powerful effect on our health, but it would be quite wrong to describe them as "concentrated" in any way. As you get into juicing and begin talking to friends about it, you will almost inevitably come across someone who'll try to warn you that too much of a good thing can be bad for you. They might cite the dimly remembered case of some health fanatic who killed himself with carrot juice. That did actually happen, but the person involved was not only drinking several gallons of fresh CJ per day, he was also guzzling toxic doses of vitamin A tablets over months and years to the point where his liver gave up on him. Obviously, he was overdoing it.

When raw juices were first discussed in medical and scientific arenas, it was suggested that they should only be taken in tiny doses, but this was undoubtedly because there wasn't a machine on the market that could easily extract juice in any quantity. Imagine what price you'd put on a glass of carrot juice if you had to grate the vegetable and somehow force it through a superfine strainer by hand. Now that we have handy centrifugal machines, the recommendation is that you must consume at least a pint of raw juice every day to begin to feel the beneficial effects.

It's true that some juices are very potent and should only be taken in small quantities. However, it will be immediately apparent to you which juices these are because they also have an intensely powerful taste and are too strong to drink straight. Juices are supposed to taste pleasant! The juices of beet and broccoli and all leafy, dark green vegetables must be diluted by at least four times the quantity of much milder juices, like carrot and apple, to be palatable.

When you first start juicing, you may well experience some slight discomfort as your body purges itself of toxins and starts to adjust, but that is transitory and to be expected. It's a good idea to start slowly, with no more than a couple of glasses of juice each day, but it is virtually impossible to overdose on raw juice. So long, that is, as you don't try to force unnatural quantities of the stuff down yourself. Drink only as much raw juice as feels comfortable, but drink as much of it as you like. There is an old adage—chew your juices and drink your foods. The juices are so delicious you may be tempted to gulp them down. Don't. It is important to drink your juices slowly, sipping them so that all their goodness is absorbed, nothing is wasted and they mix well with salivary enzymes. Then you get the biggest bang for your buck.

NEXT TO GODLINESS

Cleanliness is important with regard to the proper maintenance of your juicer, which will quickly become stained unless you take proper care of it. The strong natural pigments of the raw foods you'll be juicing will inevitably stain the plastic parts of your juicer so that you will have to soak them regularly in a bleach solution to keep your machine pristine. More importantly, you must thoroughly scour your juicer every time you use it with plenty of hot water, ensuring that the steel basket that does the work of shredding is absolutely clean and that there are no little bits of vegetable matter caught in the fine mesh of the sieve.

It's always easier to clean your juicer right after you've used it than it will be the next time you want to juice. We find that it's good practice to clean the juicer before drinking the juice we've just made. That way, we're so eager to get the chore over with that the work takes only a minute.

The Spice of Life

As you get into juicing and become accustomed to the staple combinations, you will soon lose any inhibitions you may have nurtured about tasting more pungent and increasingly earthy juices. It's important that you do. Carrot and apple or carrot and orange juices are all very good, in fact they're terrific. But to derive the maximum benefit from your juicer, it's vital that you consume as broad a variety of fruits and vegetables as possible. Leafy green vegetables are particularly important for good health, as we'll see in Chapter Nine, but they can taste foul at first. The trick is to gradually incorporate more green— more cabbage, spinach, dandelion, etc.—into your juices as you become accustomed to the taste.

Raw juices can be spiced up with the addition of root ginger, or fresh garlic, but easy does it. Both have strong flavors, which can be overpowering, and garlic in particular can have an overwhelming effect. Don't use more than one clove per glass of juice, and wash the juicer out thoroughly immediately after using garlic, otherwise the juicer is likely to become contaminated and to continue flavoring your juices for days to come. Ginger need not be peeled, just cut into cubes of about a centimeter. It can add a real zing to juices like Raw NRG (page 189).

However you choose to get into juicing, the important thing is to buy yourself a juicer and get started. Juice-making is a highly creative sport. There is always some delicious new combination just waiting to be discovered. Discover it for yourself.

4

JUICE BLITZ

"Detox" may have become a buzzword of the last few years, but it is not a recent fad. For thousands of years, mystics and shaman have used detoxification rituals in order to attain a state of heightened spirituality. Ritual fasting, with the conviction that abstinence brings us closer to God, is a feature of many religions. These days, the more privileged among us periodically spend time at health spas in order to give our battered bodies a break from rich food, poor air and the stress and strain of modern life. We hear about celebrities who seem to go in and out of clinics and detox centers without ever managing to jump off the (not so) merry-go-round of drug or alcohol addiction.

Detoxification is the process of eliminating stored wastes from the body and is the first step in curing addiction. If you are determined to give up cigarettes, for example, the Juice Blitz will help you. By consuming nothing but raw juice and spring water for 36 hours, not only will you remove the temptation to smoke after meals or over a drink, you will also facilitate the process of elimination and help to flush the nicotine out of your body. In fact, the

Juice Blitz can be a useful tool in the withdrawal stage of treatment for any form of substance abuse. Then, of course, the addict has to alter the behavioral patterns that reinforce his or her addiction.

If you don't suffer from problematic substance abuse and are not into worship, you'll still derive immense benefits from using the Juice Blitz to detoxify your system and re-focus your mind. Think of it as an internal spring clean.

Juice High

As we make our way in the world, we are profoundly affected by the negative influence of circumstances beyond our control. You can't clear the smog from the air single-handedly, or even persuade everybody to stop contributing to it by making unnecessary car trips. You can't prevent all the cruel and violent behavior that causes so much misery; you can't force your family and colleagues to treat you with respect. But there is something you can do to start taking control over your own life and destiny. You can change the quality of your health and well-being by getting rid of the toxic substances in your body and bringing yourself to a place where you are clear, calm and better able to cope with life.

If you have never, ever overindulged in any processed or chemically treated or preserved food, if you've never smoked a cigarette, done drugs or got drunk, then you probably don't need to detox your body. But how many of us have lead that kind of blameless and boring life? Bearing in mind all the junk you've put into your body over the years, you'll realize that you can't get rid of it all overnight without batting an eyelid. Like housework, the Juice Blitz takes a little effort, but the end result more than makes it all worthwhile. It's not easy to change the eating habits of a lifetime, either, but the Juice Blitz will enable you to make a fresh start.

It's too easy to allow yourself to become cynical about the state of the world around you and become so weary that you admit defeat, or lose the will to fight for what you believe in. The Juice Blitz allows you to call a stop to patterns of self-destructive behavior that undermine your health and inhibit your chances of achieving all you want from life. Its most tangible benefits include enhanced energy and stamina; people you meet who are Juice High seem to positively vibrate with life. Not only do they look good, with clear complexions and shiny hair, but they have the self-assured smile of people who know where they are going and have a pretty good idea of how to get there. We're not going to kid you that a 36-hour juice fast will enable you to become the person you always wanted to be, but we can promise that the Juice Blitz will jump start a process of transformation that could change your life.

Juice Freedom

Remember that there is nothing in raw juice that your body can't use. By going for 36 hours without consuming anything but raw juice, you will be giving your body a break and relieving it of the hard work of digestion. Left to its own devices, without having to cope with digesting food, the body will automatically initiate a full-scale house cleaning. A small minority of people finds this process uncomfortable. If you experience any of the reactions described in the "Troubleshooting" section of this chapter (page 52), take it as an indication that this cleansing process is well under way and that your body is purging itself, and be glad for that.

You may be pleasantly surprised by the effect that blitzing your body has on your mind. Many people experience an amazing mind lift almost as soon as they stop clogging their bodies with junk and start flushing their systems. Considering the synergistic relationship of the body and mind, it should be obvious that lightening the body's workload will free the mind to roam fresh horizons. The positive attitude that flows from drinking raw juice is a wonderful gift that you can use, as the shaman did, to restore internal harmony and to reconnect yourself with the universe.

Fasting on raw juices is probably the most potent short-term antidote to stress. What's more, we find that if we have a lot of work to do that requires our full concentration over long periods, it's also a great way to meet deadlines! Whenever we feel run-down and jaded, or in need of a clearer head, the Juice Blitz can not only reinvigorate our bodies, but also clear mental blockages, and help us to get a better perspective on difficult problems or vexatious situations. Sometimes we find ourselves living on nothing but raw juice for a day or two at a stretch just because it feels so good.

Crash Detox

The Juice Blitz is a crash course designed to introduce novices to the state of being Juice High. It can be performed in the comfort of your own home over the weekend if you like, since this will give you a chance for more rest. From, say, Friday night to Sunday lunchtime, all you will be putting into your body is freshly extracted raw juice. If this sounds arduous, then be reassured that you won't go hungry. Although it doesn't sit heavily in your stomach, raw juice completely satisfies the appetite. Most people find themselves perfectly happy with four to six glasses over the course of the day. However, you can drink as much as you like, so long as you don't overdo it. Have spring water too, if you like. Let your body be the judge of how much you need.

The juice recipes in this chapter demonstrate some of the classic juice combinations. They promote effective elimination and provide all the raw energy your body needs for the arduous work of deep cleansing. They are listed in the order that they should be consumed during the day, with the fruit juices to be drunk in the morning and the more savory, earthier vegetable cocktails to be taken as the day wears on. You're not required to make use of all these recipes, or even to stick to them. The recipes are highly adaptable and the possible combinations of raw juice are infinite, so feel free to improvise. But don't abandon the principle of drinking fruit juices *before* vegetable juices.

Here is what the Juice Blitz looks like:

THE NIGHT BEFORE

Start your Juice Blitz by going to bed a little hungry the night before. For dinner, drink a glass of the More Raw NRG cocktail or Potassium Punch. These are ideal, because their exceptional potassium content will counteract the acidity in your body and set up the optimum conditions for your body to do its work. Unless diluted with spring water, the root vegetable drinks may seem a little heavy for beginners to handle at this early stage in the game.

JUICE BLITZ DAY

Start the next morning with a melon or citrus juice and continue with fruit juices, which include the Sweet Sensation, until midday. For lunch, try one of the more potent vegetable cocktails, like the Beet Treat, which is a great source of sustained energy to carry you through the day. Throughout the afternoon and early evening, stick to vegetable juices in which apple is the only fruit ingredient. We find the More Raw NRG cocktail to be the most useful while detoxing, adding dark green leaves of spinach or watercress or even dandelion to increase its vitality.

Over the course of the first day of a juice fast, you may experience the odd sensation that is not entirely pleasurable. You might find yourself suddenly irritable, or tired, for instance, or you could even develop a mild headache. The best antidote to any of these symptoms is to lie down in a darkened room and take a nap. If you have been able to give over your weekend to the Juice Blitz, rest as much as possible and let your body do its work in peace. If not, rest as much as possible anyway. Don't attempt any strenuous exercise while you are blitzing, but a gentle stroll in fresh air is always a good idea.

BLITZ NIGHT AND MORNING AFTER

On Blitz night, avoid consuming anything except water after 8 o'clock. You might like to take a long, languorous bath. If you can find a friend to share it with and scrub your back, so much the better. Perhaps your friend can be persuaded to give you a massage as well. The best thing to do on Saturday night while you're Blitzing is to go to bed early and get a good night's sleep. If you're not sleepy, go to bed anyway. If you're going to bed alone, take a juicy novel or a lurid video to keep yourself entertained.

The morning after, start the day once again with fruit juice. After a good night's rest, you are likely to be feeling full of the joys of life. Even if your night was not particularly restful and you found yourself waking at dawn in a pool of sweat, you will probably feel sharper mentally. If you customarily do a crossword in the Sunday papers, we bet you'll find that you finish it faster than usual. You may also find sudden surges of energy, accompanied by some mental agitation. These are both symptoms that your metabolism has been cranked into high gear and the best antidote is a brisk walk in fresh air.

RAW ENERGY LUNCH

As you approach lunch time the second day and the end of your Juice Blitz, you may be faced with the predicament of having to sit down to a large, traditional meal or risk offending the person who cooked it. You might even be looking forward to stuffing yourself. Don't. Your first meal should be composed of at least 75 percent raw foods. That means plenty of salad.

Ease yourself back into the routine of normal meals by eating smaller portions and by taking care to chew every mouthful thoroughly. That way you will be better able to appreciate the taste of your food and it will digest more quickly.

The Rest of Your Life

Should you wish to carry on Blitzing and to continue your juice fast through the whole two days, fine. The longer you maintain your Juice Blitz, the more deep cleansing your body can accomplish at a cellular level. But don't overdo it. Your body can't reverse the negative effects of years on a poor diet in a single week, or even a month. The Juice Blitz is intended to jump-start a process that it may take years to complete; it is not a way of life. You'll know how long you can maintain a juice fast because your body will tell you when it's over by making you overwhelmingly hungry!

As soon as you experience extreme pangs of hunger, break your fast. If, at any time while Blitzing, you experience symptoms more serious than those listed in this chapter under "Troubleshooting" (page 52), consult your doctor or medical advisor. If you are contemplating a juice fast lasting longer than two or three days, it's a good idea to consult a health practitioner who is experienced in juice therapy before you begin.

Make a Plan

Before you start Blitzing, do a little planning ahead of time. You are going to need a fair quantity of fruits and vegetables, so make a list before you shop to ensure you remember everything. Where possible, always buy fruits and vegetables that have been grown organically, without the use of chemical fertilizers and pesticides. Often, organic produce doesn't look as good as the cheaper stuff that's displayed in your the supermarket, but it is inherently better for you because none of its nutritional integrity has been compromised.

Over the course of the weekend, your biggest enemy may well be boredom. Breaking from your usual dietary regime is never completely effortless, and if you are bored, you might well suffer hunger pangs and be tempted to start snacking. So find something to occupy your mind over the weekend. Read novels or watch movies; write letters or telephone friends you haven't seen for a while.

The Eight Great Eliminators

MERRY BELON

Melon goes through the system faster than any other fruit and is therefore recommended by many juice experts to be drunk on its own. They key to melon's efficacy is the exceptionally high water content of the flesh, while the nutrients are concentrated in the rind and skin, which can and should also be juiced. Some melons, like honeydew and cantaloupe, have waxy or netted skins, which can be trimmed off with a decent vegetable peeler. Others, like watermelons, can be simply scrubbed, sliced to fit your juicer and put through the machine, seeds and all.

Melons in general and watermelons in particular are a perfect source of the fluids your body needs on a daily basis and a good source of B-complex vitamins and are rich in vitamin C. There is an ever-growing profusion of melon varieties on the market, and it's fun to experiment with all of them. But melon juice can be a little on the bland side. The addition of a handful of succulent summer berries will brighten it up considerably.

Berries, those sharp little vitamin bombs, typically contain an extraordinary array of trace elements. They are the one fruit that combines really well with melons (although we're also partial to banana and melon smoothies) and the array of flavors gives lots of scope for experimentation. Try different combinations out with Merry Belon (page 185).

CITRUS ZINGER

It's well known that citrus fruits are the best sources of vitamin C, but their citric acid tends to make the juice made using a conventional conical juicer rather sharp.

Plus you get bits of pith floating in the juice that get stuck between your teeth. Whole citrus juice freshly extracted using a centrifugal machine, however, has a homogenized, creamy texture and tastes like sherbet. The bioflavonoids in the pith of citrus fruit neutralize its acidity and help the body to digest it easily. For this reason, you should always peel citrus fruit but leave on as much of the white pith as possible.

The pith of grapefruit is especially rich in bioflavonoids, which is hardly surprising since grapefruit juice tends to be the most bitter of the citrus family. Pink grapefruits are sweeter and juicier than plain yellow ones, and you have to pay a premium price for them, but it's worth it. It's sometimes hard to get hold of good, juicy oranges, but the mandarin varieties, like tangerines, are good substitutes in the depths of winter.

The skin of a citrus fruit is often waxed to preserve its shelf life and, therefore, should always be removed. Even a sliver of lemon peel put through your juicer can ruin the taste of your juice. Use lemons and limes sparingly, never adding more than half of either fruit to a glass of juice. The Citrus Zinger recipe (page 178) is a mélange of citrus spiked with ginger for an intriguing aftertaste.

FAB 5 FRUIT JUICE

In Fab 5 Fruit Juice (page 179), you can vary the fruit content as you like and depending on what you are able to buy, substituting a Clementine or Satsuma for the tangerine, white grapes for red, and pineapple, or mango for the peach. Apples and pears should be cut to fit your juicer and put through the machine, pits and all. Remove the pits from peaches and mangoes. Cut the fibrous skin from pineapples and slice them into long spears. This fruit mix is thick and frothy with a pleasant, balanced flavor that's especially good on a warm day, when you might like to add some ice cubes to it and sip it slowly through a straw.

SWEET SALVATION

Sweet bell peppers produce a juice with amazing color and fantastic flavor, but they also contain more vitamin C than oranges. Sadly, many peppers these days are grown for looks rather than flavor. Pick the ones with the deepest color and wash them well before use. Freshly made tomato juice bears little relation to the canned variety and reminds us of why these succulent, savory fruits were once called love apples. Look for vine-ripened tomatoes, which have better flavor. Sweet Salvation (page 196) has a deep red-orange color and can be a little thick. Dilute it with the judicious addition of cucumber, which should be peeled first unless it is organically grown.

MORE RAW NRG

Like the Raw NRG cocktail, More Raw NRG (page 185) is based on the crucial combination of carrot and apple, with green vegetable juices diluted by cucumber and celery. The juice extracted from green veggies is very powerful, both in its healthful properties and its taste. Spinach and watercress are invaluable for conditioning the entire digestive system thanks to the oxalic acid they contain, which helps to maintain the action of peristalsis. They are also amongst the best sources of vitamins C and E. Dandelion leaves are the first spring greens to sprout. They're an excellent source of calcium and potassium and the best-known source of beta carotene among the green vegetables. No wonder rabbits love them.

You will find the green juices a little strong at first, and will need to dilute them with cumber and celery, but as you get used to the taste you can incorporate more leaves into your juices.

POTASSIUM PUNCH

This recipe is our tribute to N. W. Walker, the raw-food pioneer and proponent of natural healing who helped to develop the technique of juicing and was the first to write about the wonders of raw juice. A marvelous testament to the truth that you are what you eat, Dr. Walker lived to the ripe old age of 106. An evangelist of detoxification, he would recommend to his patients that they drink his Raw Potassium Broth, although he would be the first to admit that most people don't find it as palatable as straight carrot juice or concoctions based on a carrot and apple mix.

The health benefits outweigh shallow considerations of taste, however. In the words of the great man himself, "The organic minerals and salts in this combination of Raw Potassium 'Broth' embrace practically the entire range of those required by the body. Its effect in reducing excessive acidity in the stomach has been truly remarkable. There is probably no food more complete in every respect than this for the human organism." So there you have it. We recommend that you drink at least a glass of Potassium Punch (page 188) a day.

BEET TREAT

You have to be careful how you handle beet juice, which is most valuable for flushing the kidneys and enriching the blood, but can cause a dramatic cleansing action if consumed in quantities of more than a half a glass at a time. Cut the fibrous roots of the bottom of your beets, but there's no need to peel them so long as they're thoroughly washed and you can include the leafy tops, too, if they are attached. Beet Treat (page 175) has a wonderful purple color and an earthy, wholesome flavor. But don't overdo it. Take it from us that too much beet juice is liable to provoke a profoundly moving experience!

ROOT SOUP

Root vegetables are the best sources of thiamin, riboflavin, niacin and other water-soluble vitamins of the B complex and are abundant in trace elements. Their juices are thick, sweet and creamy and are complemented by the slightly aniseed flavor of fennel, which adds an intriguing dimension to this recipe. Fennel is a folk cure for heartburn in the Cajun country of Louisiana and a darned effective one at that. Dilute your Root Soup (page 191) with cucumber juice, but if it's still too thick add a splash of spring water.

Brushing & Breathing

The Juice Blitz will accelerate the detoxification of your body from within by flushing the bowels and kidneys, but these are only two of the routes by which toxins are expelled. Just as important are the lungs and the skin. While detoxing, it's important to pay special attention to both.

Breathing is the most fundamental process of life. It goes without saying that if you were deprived of oxygen, you'd expire within minutes, but no less crucial is the second half of the respiratory process: discarding carbon dioxide by breathing out. CO_2 is the poisonous byproduct of oxidation and energy release in your cells, which is carried back to the lungs in the blood and eliminated when you breathe out. At least that's how it should work, but,

text continues on page 54

TROUBLESHOOTING Most people experience no discomfort while Blitzing their bodies with juice, but there are always exceptions. A small percentage of people, those whose systems are particularly toxic (and therefore most in need of detoxification) may experience one or more of the symptoms listed below. If this applies to you, don't let yourself be discouraged from continuing with the Juice Blitz for the full 36 hours. Remember that these complaints are not the signs of illness developing in your body, but of the toxins that cause illness leaving it. Recognize that they are temporary and will leave you feeling better than ever.

BLOATING AND/ OR FLATULENCE	This is quite common at the start of the Juice Blitz when you start consuming freshly extracted fruit juices on an empty stomach. Its cleansing action will sluice the walls of your stomach and stir up accumulated food debris, causing gas. Look on it as the body preparing itself for the work ahead.
DIARRHEA	What you may think of as diarrhea probably isn't and certainly should not be anything to worry about. Raw juice will wash impacted feces from your intestinal walls and expel it from the bowel in the form of loose, runny stools. This is highly beneficial and will leave you feeling lighter and renewed.
HEADACHES, MOOD SWINGS, IRRITABILITY	These are all symptomatic of the chemical change in your body and are easily overcome if you understand them as a sign that the detoxification is starting to have its effect. Take a nap, go for a walk or do the deep-breathing exercise described in this chapter.

TROUBLESHOOTING, continued	
TIREDNESS & BOREDOM	The hard work of detoxifying your body requires a lot of energy, so it's quite natural to feel sleepy. Being bored is the result of inadequate preparation. Surely you can find something to amuse yourself with? Read, watch videos, play games. Just stay out of the bar.
NASAL CONGESTION	Caught a cold, have you? Actually, a copious discharge of mucous from your nasal passage rarely indicates a viral infection but is one of the classic ways in which the body eliminates stored toxins. So blow your snotty nose and be glad you're getting rid of them.
PERSPIRATION	Your skin is the largest organ of elimination and the most direct route out of your body for a lot of toxins. Consequently, if you find that you perspire more heavily than usual while Blitzing, particularly while you're asleep in bed, don't worry about it. If you are using the Juice Blitz to stop smoking, you are liable to lose quite a lot of fluid as your body takes the opportunity to expel the nicotine through the pores of the skin.

JUICE BLITZ

THE NIGHT BEFORE

- For dinner, a glass of the More Raw NRG cocktail or Potassium Punch

JUICE BLITZ DAY

- Start with a melon or citrus juice and continue with fruit juices all day.
- Lunch: try a Beet Treat.
- Stick to vegetable juices (mixed with apple if desired) throughout the day.

since most of us use less than half of our breathing capacity, the system rarely functions as efficiently as it might. Learning to breathe properly is the most elementary step toward reconditioning your body.

Most of us breathe with only the top half of our body, but proper breathing requires the use of the diaphragm, the muscle that separates the chest cavity from the abdomen. When you breathe properly, the diaphragm contracts, allowing the lungs to expand and fill with air. During a single day, the average person will breathe in more than 11,000 liters of air. To make the best use of it all, you must learn to breathe deeply, from the bottom up. The way to best ensure proper breathing and keep your lungs working well is to make sure you get your daily dose of aerobic exercise, but taking a few minutes to perform the following deep-breathing exercise will be a great help:

1. Go outside into the fresh air or open a window.

BLITZ NIGHT & MORNING AFTER	THE REST OF YOUR LIFE
• Drink nothing but water after 8 o'clock.	• The longer you maintain the Juice Blitz the more deep-cleansing your body will do. But don't overdo it. Break your fast as soon as you experience extreme pangs of hunger.
• Start the next morning with fruit juice.	
• Lunch: plenty of salad—your first meal after the Blitz should be 75 percent raw foods.	• The Juice Blitz is a jump-start for a process that may take years to complete, it is not a way of life but an invaluable tool.

2. Stand with your feet slightly apart and your hands on your sides, touching your lower ribs just above the waist.

3. Inhale through your nose for the slow count of five and feel how your abdomen swells as you do so.

4. Continue to breathe in for another count of five, filling your lungs and expanding your rib cage.

5. Hold your breath for another count of five.

6. Exhale slowly through the mouth for a count of ten, noticing how your rib cage shrinks as you do so and pulling in with your abdominal muscles until you have expelled all the air.

7. Repeat this exercise four times.

Not only does breathing enable us to take in oxygen and expel CO_2, it also has the function of keeping the lymphatic system moving. These lymphatics are the body's sewage system: an elaborate network of microscopic channels that covers the whole body and is filled with a clear liquid called lymph. This is the medium by which nutrients are carried into the tissues of your body and metabolic waste is removed. There's more lymph in your body than blood, and the lymphatic system is similar to the tiny capillaries of the pulmonary system, but with one vital difference. Whereas blood is pumped around your body by your heart, lymph has no pump and is only kept flowing by gravity and by muscular movement.

Get Moving

One of the best techniques for encouraging lymphatic drainage and spring-cleaning your body is known as skin brushing. It stimulates the movement of interstitial fluids and breaks down congestion in areas where the flow of lymph has become sluggish. Gentle yet powerful, it takes only five minutes in the morning or evening before your bath or shower and is both invigorating and pleasurable:

1. Use a natural-fiber brush with a long handle, or a loofah.
2. Begin at the tips of your shoulders and cover your whole body (except the head), working downward, with long, smooth strokes over the shoulders, arms and trunk.
3. Starting at the feet, brush upward over the legs and hips.

You need only go over your skin once for the brushing to be effective. Regular brushing will stimulate lymph-flow and unclog the pores of your skin. How firmly you press depends entirely on how well toned your skin is. Go easy to begin with, and become more vigorous as your skin gets healthier.

5

BODY BUILDING

Juice drinking works two kinds of magic on your body. The first is detoxification. It clears out spaces in your body that other foods just can't reach. And detox is central not only to healing illness but to protecting the body from degeneration as well as regenerating and rejuvenating it. That is why it forms the basis of every form of natural medicine in the world. The principle is simple: Clean out the body and you raise its vitality, strengthen its healing powers and set it free of the burden of chronic fatigue and heaviness that plagues the majority of men and women in industrialized counties these days. Once, detox itself was probably enough to heal and boost vitality. Now, as a result of widespread nutritional deficiencies, it is only half of what is called for. Now we need to look not only at how to *detox* the system but how to *rebuild* its metabolic pathways. We call this process body building.

Get a Life

As a result of the way we have depleted our foods of essential nutrients and distorted the vitamin and mineral balance in our bodies through chemical farming, heavy food processing and long storage of our foods, most of us these days have nowhere near the optimal levels of vitamins, minerals and vital trace elements our bodies need to be superhealthy. And while you can survive for a time without them, you cannot live at a high level of well-being. Many nutrients— from vitamin B6 to the mineral zinc and the trace element silicon—must be present both in adequate amounts and in a good balance in order for the enzymes on which every life process, whether it be the building of new cell walls, the formation of hormones in the body, or the digestion and assimilation of food, depends. Minerals and trace elements are especially important.

Your body cannot make its own minerals. It has to take them in, in a good balance, from the foods you eat. In addition to nitrogen, potassium and phosphorus, to stay healthy, the body requires magnesium, manganese and calcium, selenium, zinc, copper, iodine, boron, molybdenum, vanadium and probably other elements as yet undiscovered. These elements need to come from the foods you eat. Generally they do when foods are grown organically in healthy, traditionally fertilized soils. But they are increasingly missing and unbalanced in the foods we buy today thanks to our legacy of chemical farming.

ORGANIC MAGIC

The organic matter in healthy soil is nature's factory for biological activity. It is built up as a result of the breakdown of vegetable and animal matter by the soil's natural "residents"—worms, bacteria and other useful microorganisms. The presence of these creatures in the right quantity and types gives rise to physical, chemical and biological properties that create fertility in our soils and make plants grown on them highly resistant to disease.

When it comes to human health, they do a lot more. The minerals and trace elements we need to trigger the metabolic processes on which the manufacture of hormones in the body, as well as over all health, depends must be in an organic form. That is, they need to be taken from living things like plant or animal foods. You cannot eat nails—inorganic iron—for instance, and expect to protect yourself from anemia, or chew sand—inorganic silica—and be sure to get enough of the trace element to keep your nails and hair strong and help protect your bones from osteoporosis. It is the organic matter in soil that enables plants to transform inorganic iron and silica into the organic form which is taken up by the vegetables and fruits, grains and legumes grown on the soil. When we eat that produce, these nutrients become available to our bodies. Destroy the soil's organic matter through chemical farming—which is just what we have done in the past 75 years—and slowly but inexorably you destroy the health of people and animals living on foods grown on it. Organic methods of farming help protect against significant distortions in mineral balances—that is from an increase in one or more mineral elements that can alter the availability of others and undermine health. No such protection is available when foods are chemically grown.

Making Do

Your body has a remarkable ability to compensate for a mineral or trace element missing from your food. But, as a result of many years of our having eaten nutritionally depleted foods, multiple deficiencies have become widespread. According to large-scale studies, few people in the West now get all the minerals they need to ensure that the metabolic processes work adequately—processes on which health, energy and the immune system depend. The deficiencies we are developing have brought metabolic distortions in their wake—such as degenerative diseases, early aging and emotional disturbances like depression and anxiety. These kinds of deficiencies cannot easily be corrected. Popping the latest multimineral tablet from your corner pharmacy or health food store won't do it. Daily juicing will.

For nutrients in foods exist in complex synergy and affect each other. They also interact and work together in your body. The balance of bio-available minerals and trace elements needed in the body for peak well-being, like the balance available from wholesome foods, is infinitely more complex than vitamin fanatics would have us believe. This is where raw juices really come into their own. To restore biochemical balance once it has been disturbed, you need a continual supply of the vitamins and minerals as well as other, as yet unidentified, health enhancing substances that are found in fresh vegetables and fruits—usually also supplemented with extra green plants such as seaweeds, spirulina, chlorella, barley grass or alfalfa. Drinking fresh juices daily can restore metabolic balance and eliminate deficiencies faster than anything else.

Perfect Synergy

Some of the most valuable of the new nutritional disciplines is research involved in seeking out and identifying specific nutrients and compounds—called phytochemicals—present within common foods which are natural cancer and other disease preventers. In recent years, some fascinating studies have been undertaken to identify the substances and compounds locked within them that give them their power. Thanks to the particular balance of amino acids, enzymes, polysaccharides and other compounds they contain, such foods as garlic, licorice and green compounds like green barley, spirulina, chlorella, licorice, as well as many other fresh foods, often have the ability to turn on the human immune system. Many are capable of stimulating T-cell and B-cell production. Some contain isoflavones and protease inhibitors, which are capable of breaking down layers surrounding foreign proteins including tumors. Others are rich in phytosterols, which are useful in protecting both men and women from the reproductive damage by herbicides and pesticides that act as estrogen-mimics—lowering sperm count in men and encouraging PMS, osteoporosis, endometriosis and fibroids in women. In recent years a number of international conferences have been organized to examine the properties of these so called "designer foods."

NARROW-MINDED NUTRITION

One of the problems with most of the information that is handed out through the media and books on nutrition is that it is highly fragmented. You hear talk about a specific vitamin or mineral and how we should take more of it, about cholesterol or protein or fiber. We seem to have become obsessed in recent years with breaking everything down and looking at the effects of specific ingredients on our bodies. This has created a situation in which we have forgotten how to see the forest for the trees. We have forgotten that it is not just the ingredient—a particular vitamin or mineral or compound—in a vegetable, for instance, that can do us good. It is the synergy of nature in which the whole is far greater than the sum of its parts, even if scientists were intelligent enough to isolate each and study it. What we lack is an awareness of the total benefit of fresh foods in their ability to strengthen the immune system, to protect us against acute illness such as flus and colds as well as long term degenerative conditions like cancer, arthritis and coronary heart disease, to rejuvenate our bodies and to help us reach our full potential mentally, physically and spiritually.

PROTECTIVE COMPOUNDS

Many phytochemicals in fresh vegetables are known to have cancer-preventing properties. They come in a total package in fresh fruits and vegetables and work together in perfect synergy so that the whole is far greater than any of its parts. Recent research carried out into the soybean's health-giving phytochemicals has produced a growing list of specific ingredients, each of which has something important to offer. Some of the most important are these:

SAPONINS These have antioxidant properties and as such help prevent changes to the cells' DNA associated with premature aging and the development of cancer. Research shows that cancer of the colon is much lower in populations where there is a high dietary intake of saponins.

PHYTOSTEROLS These plant hormones include such chemicals as stigmasterol and ergosterol which are little absorbed in the digestive system. They pass on to the colon where they help prevent damage from the cancer-producing breakdown products from cholesterol. Some phytosterols are also weak estrogenic compounds capable of binding with estrogen receptor sites in both male and female bodies, protecting against reproductive problems that develop as a result of exposure to xenestrogens. Many also help protect against premature aging of the skin and skin cancer as well as prostate troubles, PMS and menopausal miseries.

PHENOLIC ACIDS These antioxidants help prevent damage to cellular DNA associated with premature aging and the development of degenerative diseases.

PROTEASE INHIBITORS These compounds help protect against the damaging effects of toxins in the body and against radiation and free-radical damage. In laboratory studies, protease inhibitors have been shown to inhibit cancers of the mouth, pancreas, lung, colon and digestive tract. Unfortunately, protease inhibitors—which exist in good quantities in many common wholesome foods, including potatoes, eggs and grains—are greatly destroyed by cooking. In many raw vegetables, however, they are in rich supply.

OMEGA-3 FATTY ACIDS These are essential fatty acids that, when unadulterated by heating or processing and taken fresh, have been shown to protect against cancer and heart disease. They also play important roles in the manufacture of hormones in the body and are found in good quantities in flaxseed oil or flaxseeds, in sprouted seeds and grains that you can use for juicing, and in some of the special green foods such as spirulina.

ISOFLAVONES These are plant hormones which carry strong anticancer properties particularly in relation to cancers of the reproductive system such as prostate cancer, cervical cancer, ovarian cancer, endometrial cancer and breast cancer. A lot of research into the effects of isoflavones has also been done in animal studies. The molecular structure of isoflavinoids is very close to that of the estrogens, however their estrogenic actions on the body—

unlike the dangerous petro-chemically derived estrogen-mimics or *xenestrogens* in the environment—are very weak. In fact, they are only a 100-thousandth as potent as the body's estrogens and estrogens given in the form of drugs. Eating foods or making juices from foods rich in the isoflavones can help protect both men and women from estrogens in the environment. Japanese researchers have shown that the isoflavones, with their weak estrogenic effects, can relieve—often even completely eliminate—the negative symptoms associated with PMS and menopause.

Plant compounds are important in the body-building process. They too play an important, if not yet fully understood, part in restoring the kind of biochemical balance that the body's metabolic processes need to function smoothly. They work in perfect synergy with the vitamins, minerals and trace elements which occur with them in the fresh unprocessed fruits and vegetables you make your juices from. You need only examine a couple of common vegetables to see just how mind-blowing the protective, restoring plant compounds they contain can be.

KING CARROT

Take the carrot. Carrots are unbelievably rich in antioxidant- and cancer-preventative compounds, especially the carotinoids. The most well-known is beta carotene. This naturally occurring antioxidant has become famous in recent years as a safe-to-take precursor to vitamin A—something that your body can turn into vitamin A as needed. But beta carotene is only the most well researched of the carotinoids. Scientists are now discovering that there are also many others that appear to have equal, if not greater, health-supporting abilities. The link between these carotinoids and disease prevention has now been well established in scientific literature. A high consumption of foods containing them has been shown to lower the incidence of lung, pancreas and prostate cancer, for instance. Even cancer among cigarette smokers is lower among people with carotinoid-rich diets. So much is this true that smokers on carotinoid-poor diets are four times more likely to get cancer than those who consume the carotinoids in even one carrot a day. Think how much more you get when you drink a full glass of fresh carrot juice each day. But the carotinoids are by no means the only goodies in carrot juice. Nor are carrots the only place that you will find good quantities of them. Spirulina—which is a wonderful green additive to juices—is ultrarich in carotinoids; other vegetables such as winter squash and yams are equally rich as carrots. So are many of the green vegetables from cabbage to beet tops (see Green Lightning, page 146).

The glory of the carrot and the beauty of juice made from it is that it contains over 40 known protective and cancer-preventative compounds for protection, regeneration and rejuvenation, in addition to all of the wonderful minerals and vitamins tucked into this inexpensive and delicious root veggie. Carrots also contain other fabulous health-boosting friends such as MOP, which is short for methoxypsoralen, a little compound with an amazing ability to help repair DNA. DNA is the blueprint of life carried in the cells. When DNA remains intact, as cells replicate the new cells are born perfect. However all those things that cause free-radical damage—from chemicals in our food or water or air to exposure to the ultraviolet rays of the sun—can damage DNA so that as cells reproduce they no longer resemble the original cell from which they came. Instead they become twisted and distorted versions of it and are unable to function normally. Damage to DNA is the central cause of degeneration and premature aging in the body. Prevent it and you can prevent early aging. That is where MOP comes in. MOP actually tucks itself in between the base pairs of DNA molecules and repairs damage that has occurred. Scientists experimenting with MOP have found that they can take damaged white blood cells from people, add MOP to them and then put the white blood cells back into the body in perfect shape. Parsnips are also rich in MOP and mix well with carrot juice.

GREEN GLORY

When you look at what is in the humble broccoli, again all sorts of fascinating stuff turns up that can do you so much good that you end up wondering why you have been feeding on processed foods for so long. There are an amazing 33 cancer-preventive compounds in fresh broccoli. Things

CANCER PREVENTATIVE COMPOUNDS FOUND IN BROCCOLI		
beta carotene	iso-phenyl-ethyl-thiocyanate	salicylic acid
beta sitosterol	kaempferol	sinapic acid
caffeic acid	linoleic acid	sinigrin
chlorogenic acid	oleracea demutagenic factor brassica	squalene
chlorophyll	para-coumaric acid	stigmasterol
cinnamic acid	para-hydroxy benzoic acid	succinic acid
cycloartanol 42-methylene	phytic acid	trans ferulic acid
ferulic acid	protein (brassica oleracea)	vanillic acid
indole-3-acetonitrile	quercetin	vitamin C
indole-3-carbinol	quercetrin	3-3-di-methane indoxyl
iso-allyl-thiocyanate	rutin	

like beta carotene and indole-3-carbinol have the ability to counteract many of the chemicals that pollute our environment such as the nitrosamines that are known to cause cancer. Nitrosamines are formed when nitrites are used to preserve and color meat. And compounds like indole-3-carbinol—which render destructive chemicals unable to cause damage to the body—not only prevent cancer, they also help prevent other degenerative diseases as well as premature aging. They also help regenerate and rejuvenate your body. A cup full of broccoli or one of the other dark greens in a glass of carrot and apple juice once a day promises 165 percent of the recommended daily allowance for vitamin C, 40 percent for vitamin A and 20 percent for calcium. To give you some idea of just how powerful the protective properties of green can be, below is a list of the *known* cancer preventive compounds in broccoli.

Most people have never heard of the indoles or saponins or any of the other fresh food compounds that can encourage radiant health, although volumes have been written about their virtues in scientific literature. But even more esoteric is the knowledge about how juices made from fresh raw foods enhance health not from a *chemical* point of view but rather from an *energetic* one. To begin to understand that, you have to turn to some of the world experts in natural healing who have made remarkable use of them to do everything from helping the body eliminate cancer from its system, curing migraines, rejuvenating, and improving athletic performance. Raw foods and the juices you make from them do some pretty amazing things.

Back to Basics

Human evolution is a slow process. For hundreds of generations, our ancestors lived on wild foods gathered and eaten raw. Our genes appear to be specially adapted to dealing with raw foods. This may be the reason why they have been used for generations by experts in natural medicine, such as the famous Swiss physician Max Bircher-Benner and the German Max Gerson, not only to support the human organism's healing but also to heighten vitality as well as to regenerate and rejuvenate the body as a whole. There are mysterious health-promoting qualities in living foods that nutritional science is only just beginning to investigate and will certainly never really penetrate until it breaks out of its blinkered reliance on the chemistry of food's interactions with the body alone. Meanwhile, incorporating a good percentage of live foods—fresh vegetables, raw seeds and nuts, fresh sprouted grains and seeds, and especially fresh vegetable juices—in your diet can help rebalance hormones, stabilize moods, clear and rejuvenate skin, shed excess fat stores and transform your emotional and spiritual outlook on life.

More than 50 years ago, Hans Eppinger, chief doctor at the First Medical Clinic of the University of Vienna, discovered that eating raw foods leads to increased cellular respiration. It does this in a number of ways, by creating a kind of positive feedback loop, where one thing in turn stimulates another until cell metabolism is heightened. It eliminates accumulated wastes and toxins from cells and tissues. It supplies the level of nutrients essential for optimal cell function. And, perhaps most important of all, it heightens the micro-electrical tensions associated with cell vitality so that even cells in a particularly sluggish and neglected system are revitalized. They become better able to burn calories in the presence of oxygen and to produce energy efficiently both for overall vitality and for carrying out the housekeeping on which the health of your body depends.

MICROELECTRICS

Capillaries are minute blood vessels which form the vast network of microcirculation throughout your body. It is their responsibility to deliver oxygen-rich blood for it to be used by the cells. So important are these fine vessels that nature has supplied you with incredible lengths of them. If you were to attach all the capillaries in your body end to end, they would measure some 60,000 miles in length—more than twice around the world. The state of your capillaries depends to a great extent the condition of your body as a whole, for they are the arbitrators of cell nutrition, respiration and elimination. It is through these capillaries that nutrients and oxygen are carried. Each of them has tiny "pores" that allow plasma but not red blood cells to seep through and pass into the body fluid. This is how nutrients are delivered and wastes eliminated from tissues. Without a good microcirculation, metabolism cannot take place efficiently. That is why the capillaries play a vital part in the successful elimination of excess fat deposits with all their stored toxins.

Unfortunately, over the years, the capillaries of people living on the average Western diet—with its excessive fats, proteins and refined and processed foods—become twisted, distended and highly porous. When they do, proteins seep through and deposit themselves between the tissues and the capillary walls, where they interfere with proper oxygen exchange and impede nutrient delivery and waste elimination. This can gradually starve cells, tissues and organs of all they need to function properly and can also lower cellular metabolic activity. Such changes in microcirculation lower overall vitality because the body's tissues are not receiving the oxygen and nutrients they need for healthy metabolic functions. In this deprived condition, the entire organism (i.e., your body) is predisposed to degenerative illness and rapid aging. A Juice High lifestyle, drinking three or four glasses of freshly made juice a day, at least two of which are primarily vegetable juices, helps restore normal microcirculation. This heightens metabolism, keeping your weight down and maintaining a high level of energy, and, in a very real way, it also rejuvenates your body.

DYNAMIC TENSIONS

The interchange of chemicals and energy between the microcirculation and the cells takes place through two thin membranes and a fine interstitial space. It happens only because the cells and capillaries have what is known as "selective capacity." This means they are able to absorb the substances they need and to reject what is harmful or unnecessary for metabolic processes. This selective capacity is the result of antagonist chemical and micro-electrical tensions in the cells and tissues of all living systems. When you die, these microelectrical tensions are lost completely. When you suffer from a chronic degenerative condition or when metabolism is lowered, they are drastically reduced. The stronger the tensions, the more intense these antagonisms, the healthier and more vital your body will be and the more efficiently it will be able to burn off stored fat and eliminate toxicity. The chronic fatigue and lowered metabolism that typically occur in women as they grow older— particularly if they have been on and off low-calorie diets over the years—is accompanied by a decrease in chemical and micro-electrical tensions and a loss in selective capacity. This situation in turn leads to a lowering of cell metabolism and to a slowing down of cell reproduction. It can also result in a weakening of the capillary walls and in the gradual build-up in the interstitial spaces of a sticky "marsh" derived from excess waste products. This marsh, or tissue sludge, impedes biochemical processes (including the production and balancing of hormones) and tends to lower metabolism even further, impairing the efficient elimination of wastes by the lymph system.

This opalescent liquid carries the waste and toxic products from these minute channels into larger lymphatic vessels, on through the lymph nodes, which are located in the groin and under the arm and the neck. The lymph nodes filter the fluid to remove impurities and dead cells; they are also a place where antibodies, which fight infection or toxins, are made. After purification at the nodes, the fluid is returned to the blood. However, when the lymph system becomes clogged or does not eliminate properly, the body can become seriously burdened with toxicity.

It is the common factor in the development of degenerative diseases such as arthritis, cancer, heart disease and diabetes as well as early aging and even the development of persistent cellulite in women's bodies and in the tendency to store and to maintain a high level of fat deposits in both men and women.

Meet Selective Capacity

Eppinger and another German scientist, Karl Eimer, showed why drinking live juices and eating lots of fresh raw vegetables can change all this. They steadily *increase* selective capacity by heightening electrical potentials between tissue cells and capillary blood. This improves the ability of your capillaries to regulate the transport of nutrients. It also helps detoxify the system, removing any sticky marsh of waste products present. Together with exercise, a way of eating a lot of living foods and their juices—where roughly 50 percent of what you eat is raw—breaks through that vicious circle of fatigue and relying on coffee, sugar and chocolate just to keep going, replacing it with a high-functioning metabolism which makes detoxification and the rebuilding of the body's vitamins, minerals, trace elements and enzymic systems on which good metabolism depends a steady, straightforward occurrence.

Drink lots of raw juices and choose the rest of your foods from wholesome, natural products such as grains and legumes, tofu, sea plants and fresh, locally grown vegetables and fruits, and you will notice a dramatic improvement in how you look and feel and function within the first couple of weeks. But it will be several weeks before the burden of toxicity which you have been carrying has fully cleared, and it will probably be a few months before even deeper benefits begin to show themselves. By then any pre-existing subclinical vitamin or mineral deficiencies are cleared up completely. But be patient. Your body has a quite magnificent ability to heal itself and to excel at being superhealthy, but this doesn't happen overnight.

6

THE HIGH LIFE DIET

The Juice Blitz is a first-rate, quick-fix detox regime that gives you an intimation of the Juice High lifestyle. Once you've experienced its clear-headed benefits, you'll want to take it further. The next step is *body building*, using raw juices to replenish lost vitamins, mineral and trace elements, as well as unidentified factors that help prevent degenerative diseases as well as energize, regenerate and rejuvenate your body. The High Life Diet will give you all the support you need to take this step.

This is an exciting, delicious food style for the future, which satisfies the senses and fuels the body so that it functions at peak efficiency on an ongoing basis. Its high raw-food content and its dependence on wholesome *real* food—instead of the ersatz packaged stuff that masquerades as food—provides the kind of high-quality nutrition you require to feel fully alive. At the end of this chapter, we give you ten days' worth of recipes which can be followed as a short-term, quick-fix regime to enhance your overall health. More significantly, it can be used as the blueprint for a permanent change in the way you eat to build and sustain optimum well-being.

The Big Idea

There is nothing complicated about the High Life—just a few simple principles that determine what to eat and when to eat it. Breakfast is raw juice with green supplements and as much whole fruit as you want. Try to make lunch the main meal of the day. It begins with a green drink and is built around a terrific Trio Salad (see page 92) composed of one root vegetable, one fruit vegetable and one leafy vegetable, or another seductive salad of your choice. What else? A good source of protein such as tofu, eggs, steamed or grilled fish or chicken—preferably cooked without the skin—and organic meat.

Dinner should be light. Perhaps a glass of raw juice followed by a bowl of homemade vegetable soup spiked with sea vegetables for extra minerals and flavor, or a crunchy salad with some whole-grain bread. Lunch and dinner are interchangeable. It may not be practicable for you to take a long break in the middle of the day, but whenever possible make lunch your largest meal. This is when you most need energy for the day. If you get into the habit of eating light in the evening, you'll find that you will sleep far better at night.

Soon, you will probably find that you are sleeping a lot less, too. When your body is detoxified and functioning efficiently, you will sleep more soundly. Because the sleep you get on the High Life Diet is more restful, you need less of it.

CUT OUT COFFEE

We love coffee, adore the stuff. The kind of coffee we particularly like is really strong, dark and potent espresso of the kind that gives you a better buzz than amphetamine sulphate. The comparison with an illegal drug is apposite since trimethyl xanthine—caffeine—is also habit-forming, and its overuse can lead to headaches, insomnia, nervousness and anxiety. Like speed, coffee gives you a quick lift and the illusion of energy, only to let you crash a few hours later in need of another caffeine injection to keep going. Consequently, while we still drink coffee occasionally, we're careful not to let it become a daily habit.

Have you ever had to work late, perhaps studying for an exam, and kept yourself going with endless cups of coffee? If so, you'll be familiar with that wired mental state in which your thoughts are racing but you just can't seem get to them into any sort of comprehensible order. Caffeine stimulates your nervous system and makes you feel alert, but tests have demonstrated that in reality the drug causes confusion and nervousness. Rather than help you concentrate, too much coffee has the effect of disconnecting you from your instincts and, in extreme cases, can provoke a psychotic reaction. In fact, if you need a clear head and the stamina to keep studying for hours on end, the best thing to keep you going is a glass of raw juice.

Some people use coffee as a laxative, but while it's certainly effective at moving the bowels, caffeine has a strongly adverse effect on the digestive system as a whole. Tea is not much better for you. Even if you've always been a committed tea drinker, after a couple of weeks of living the High Life you'll find you don't miss it. Then, you will appreciate an occasional cup of English Breakfast or powerful shot of espresso as one of life's simple pleasures rather than a matter of addiction.

TABLE MANNERS

Eating and drinking are usually seen as correlated activities. We tend to do both at meal times, simultaneously sluicing chewed food down our esophagus with abandon while raising the next forkful to our lips. Too often we eat on the run, cramming food into our mouths and washing it down with great gulps of drink. We know that eating like this isn't very dignified and probably isn't too good for the digestion, but we do it anyway. Then, when we get indigestion, we complain that there must have been something wrong with the food rather than the way we consumed it.

To live the High Life, however, you are going to have to do something about sloppy table manners. The High Life Diet requires you to become more discriminating about what you eat, but you must also be more fastidious about the way you eat it. While we occasionally enjoy a glass of wine or two over dinner, drinking a lot at meal times is not a good idea for two reasons. First, drinking tends to make you chew your food less thoroughly than you should. Second, fluids dilute the saliva in your mouth and the gastric juices in your stomach, rendering them ineffective at breaking down the improperly chewed food.

Accompany your meals with a glass of spring water if you wish, but just the one. Sip it slowly between mouthfuls, to clear your palate. Take the time to chew your food thoroughly before swallowing it. Don't talk with your mouth full and don't leap up from the table as soon as you're finished, but take a calm minute to let your food settle.

JUST JUICE

You'll notice how a glass of raw juice tends to fill you up, as if it were a meal in itself. In fact, considering the nutritional value of raw juice, it is a meal in itself and should be consumed on its own. Raw juice is easy to digest, but it still has to pass through your stomach to be assimilated in your intestines, and anything eaten at the same time will only slow its passage. If taken on an empty stomach, raw juice will take no more than 20 minutes to pass through your stomach. Therefore, make it a rule not to eat or drink anything for at least that length of time after downing a glass of raw juice.

The living enzymes in raw juice assist the digestion process and the neutralizing effect of raw juice upon the internal environment of your body will provide the ideal conditions for food to be properly digested. Consequently, raw juice makes the ideal aperitif, or first course of a meal. At dinner parties, your guests will be delighted and amazed by being offered a glass of freshly extracted raw juice in place of soup. Just remember (and tell your friends!) to sip your juice slowly, mixing it with the saliva in your mouth, and wait half an hour whenever you can before moving on to the main course.

With fruit juices, the half hour rule is slightly different, but even more important. Fruit juices pass through your stomach really quickly, in 10 or 15 minutes, so long as there is no food in the way. If the exit to your intestines is blocked by half-digested food, the fruit juice will be trapped in your stomach where it will start to ferment, causing bloating and flatulence. For this reason, fresh fruit and fruit juices should only be consumed on an empty stomach.

In Chapter Three, we explained why fruit juices are the best things to put into your body in the morning, because they are easily digested and offer instant energy in the form of natural sugar. In learning to live the High Life, take that principle further by resolving to consume nothing but freshly extracted fruit juices right up until midday. This will allow your body to complete its work of elimination before you start to burden your system once more with food and, as such, could well be the smartest move you ever make.

ONE GREEN GLASS

Fruit juices are fabulous, naturally, and we have yet to meet someone who wasn't beguiled by their first taste of Carrot & Apple. These are the easiest juices to accept, but they are far from being the most beneficial. In Chapter Nine, we explain more about the amazing and as yet unidentified health-promoting factors in the juices of green, leafy vegetables that have an awesome power to combat disease and to condition the body. To really live the High Life, you must incorporate more green vegetables into your diet. That's not a radical statement; everybody is it saying it, from government agencies to your mother.

To derive the maximum benefit from your juicer, you must make full use of the pungent and powerfully-flavored dark green juices extracted from such vegetables as spinach, broccoli and cabbage. These all contain an abundance of micronutrients, enzymes and trace elements that are easily denatured by heat and totally destroyed by cooking. By juicing them, we are able to extract most of the essential goodness of raw vegetables and supply our bodies with unadulterated, natural green nutrition.

The catch is that these green juices tend to be something of an acquired taste. They are too strong to be drunk straight and must be diluted with blander and more watery salad vegetables, like cucumber and celery. Cucumbers are rich in minerals but are mostly water; the juice is a strong diuretic and the best skin toner we know of. Unfortunately, the bright green specimens you see in the supermarket have often been sprayed with pesticides and waxed to preserve their appeal. Unless you're sure your cuke is organic, peel it. Celery has a mildly salty flavor and is also good for the complexion. It's often a little muddy at the root, so wash each stalk thoroughly before you put it through the juicer.

Make it a rule that you will drink at least one glass of green juice each day. That doesn't mean you have to stick exclusively to green ingredients, just make sure that they form a good percentage of what you juice. Use a base of carrot and apple, as we do in the Raw NRG mix (see page 189) and gradually include more and more green, as in the More Raw NRG cocktail (see page 185). Generally speaking, the darker green the color of your juice, the more good it's going to do you. See Chapter Nine for a more thorough discussion of Green Lightning and for advice on green supplements like spirulina and green barley, which can be added to raw juice to increase its green quotient.

GO ORGANIC

The quality of the produce that we can buy most easily and cheaply is not all it should be. In Chapter Nine, we discuss in more detail the reasons why buying organic produce where possible is always the best policy. Produce that has been grown without the use of artificial fertilizers and chemical pesticides is inherently healthier than plants that have been subjected to the battery of modern farming methods. Organically grown fruit and vegetables may not look so big and shiny, but they retain their nutritional integrity and do not contain chemical residues.

Organic produce is more expensive than conventional, but worth paying the premium for. If you can't find an organic green grocer locally, perhaps there is a produce cooperative or CSA-box program operating in your neighborhood. If not, perhaps you'd like to start one. See the Resources section for details of how to find organic food outlets near you.

LESS IS MORE
Busy people tend to skip meals. They get caught up in their work, rushing to meet deadlines, and neglect to eat. This is by no means a bad thing, since being slightly hungry tends to make us more alert and creative. In fact it would be fine if, once their work was done, these busy people took their time to prepare and consume a properly-balanced meal like the ones we suggest in the recipe section below. But busy people don't tend to do that. They're too busy. So they live on convenience food.

People who want to lose weight in a hurry also tend to skip meals. They figure that by doing without lunch they can forgo a few calories and maybe shed a few ounces. It might work, too, except that too often they find themselves craving sweets in the middle of the afternoon, or being irresistibly drawn to the soft drink machine in the corner of the office. There's nothing wrong with skipping meals, so long as you don't try to compensate for the meal you missed by eating (or drinking) junk later on.

Not only is there nothing wrong with skipping meals, it can be positively good for you. Increasingly, scientific evidence suggests that longevity can be significantly increased by a diet that contains a high level of essential nutrients, but about a third fewer calories than are conventionally thought necessary to maintain "normal" body weight. A glass of raw juice is the ultimate dietary supplement and the perfect replacement for a bulky meal because it is nutrient-dense, but calorie-lean. Have a glass of raw juice instead of lunch and you will probably have plenty of energy to last you through until late afternoon. If you miss lunch and come home starving, don't dive into the cookie jar or raid the fridge for something to snack on before dinner. Make yourself a glass of raw juice instead.

WHERE'S THE FIBER?

Nutritionally, raw juice is excellent, but it is totally deficient in one department. Of all the insoluble fiber contained within the fruits and vegetables you juice, none of it goes into the glass. It's precisely because all the fiber has been extracted that raw juice is so effective in delivering essential nutrients to the body, but mankind cannot live by juice alone. Plenty of fiber in your diet is a prerequisite for good health and proper elimination, because it provides the muscles in your digestive tract something solid to work with and acts as a peristaltic broom, collecting fecal matter in your colon and propelling it to the bowels. Fiber, as they say, keeps you regular.

The best source of fiber is raw fruits and vegetables, whole grains and pulses, of which you'll find plenty in the High Life Diet. Raw juice does contain some soluble dietary fiber, but all the insoluble cellulose fiber ends up with the pulp. We're frequently asked what to do with the pulp left over from juicing and there are various ways in which it can be used.

Pulp Facts and Pulp Fiction

One of the big mistakes many of the books on juicing make is they don't tell you what to do with the pulp. The pulp is important. The high fiber present in natural fruits and vegetables has a very low caloric density but usually lots of flavor. Since the average person on a Western diet gets only 10 to 25 grams of fiber a day, where our ancestors were used to 35 to 60 grams a day, the more fiber you can use from your juicing, the better. There are even some experts that have come to believe that the decrease in our intake of plant fiber we have witnessed in the last 50 years may be enough to account for the rampant degenerative conditions that have developed in our societies.

There are all sorts of things you can do with vegetable and fruit pulps, but there is one principle you have to know. Either use it right away in whatever dish you want to make—salad, sorbet, meatloaf, sauce, or a poultice (more about this in a minute)—or freeze it. It is easy to freeze fruit and vegetable pulps in plastic bags that you can then take out and use at your leisure for whatever purposes you want.

CHEAP BEAUTY

From a health and good looks point of view, there are all sorts of wonderful external poultices you can make from vegetable and fruit pulps. The pulp of kiwifruit, pineapple, papaya and mango are wonderful for refining skin—in fact, they are the natural source of the AHA fruit acids that you pay a fortune for in expensive skin creams these days. Simply apply the pulp to your skin, leave it on for ten minutes and rinse it off. Because these tropical fruits contain proteolytic enzymes they will quite literally digest the dead skin cells on the surface of your skin, leaving it smoother, fresher and regenerated.

The pulp from potatoes and cucumber are very useful as eye compresses. Simply place between two pieces of cheesecloth or cotton and lay over the lids of closed eyes while you rest for 10 or 15 minutes. It takes away black circles and bags from under the eyes.

Pumpkin, cucumber, carrot and squash pulps are great for calming skin inflammations, whether it be eczema, rash or sunburn. They are very cooling to the body and can be very useful when you have a mild fever. Place the pulp in a compress in between two pieces of cotton on the forehead or just over the liver.

Pulps make great additions to salads too. You can also use pulp to stuff zucchinis, tomatoes, squash, even twice-baked potatoes (bake a potato, take out the inner part of the potato, mix with vegetable pulp, season with salt, pepper, and a little olive oil. Put them back in the oven sprinkled with some chopped green onions and rebake for 15 minutes.) Pulp also does well in pasta salads. Also, you can make wonderful soups by juicing vegetables then mixing some of the juice back into the pulp and eating it immediately.

DELICIOUS SWEETS

You can use the pulp of fruits to bake beautiful sweet breads and rolls or make carrot cake. Fruit pulp, fresh or frozen, such as apricot, pear, apple and peach, also is a great thing to add to porridge, granola or cereals along with a dash of cinnamon, nutmeg or cardamom. It brings a natural sweetness to the cereal without you ever having to add honey or sugar. You can also mix fruit pulp with yogurt, cottage cheese or tofu, adding a little unsulphured blackstrap molasses or maple syrup to make delicious shakes. Finally, you can use fruit pulps warmed up a little to make delicious toppings for toast, pancakes or muffins. You can even mix it in with minced lamb or beef, pork or chicken, to make delicious high-fiber patties. Any pulp left over that you don't have a use for makes fabulous compost. You don't even have to wait for it to rot down, just spread it around your garden.

Here are a few of our favorite recipes, but do develop your own. You would be surprised how much you can get out of pulp.

Coleslaw

2 cups cabbage pulp
2 cups carrot pulp
1 cup apple pulp
1 tbsp cider vinegar
3 tbsp olive oil
2 tbsp chopped parsley
chopped green onions

Mix all of the pulp together, stir in the vinegar and olive oil, and garnish with the parsley and spring onion.

Pasta Salad

1 bag whole-grain pasta of your choice
3 tbsp carrot pulp
3 tbsp celery pulp
3 tbsp tomato pulp
3 tbsp cauliflower pulp
salt and pepper to taste
1 tsp oregano
2 garlic cloves, pressed

4 tbsp olive oil

Cook the pasta and chill. Add the rest of the ingredients, mix and serve.

Yummy Carrot Cake

1 cup cold-pressed sesame oil or olive oil

3 cups carrot pulp

1 cup apple pulp

1/2 cup blackstrap molasses

1 cup honey

3 eggs

3 cups whole-grain flour

1 tsp baking soda

1 tsp pure vanilla extract

1 cup raisins

2 tsp nutmeg

Mix the pulps together, add the honey, molasses, vanilla and eggs and mix together well. Sift together the dry ingredients and add to the mixture. Stir until blended. Add the raisins, pour into an oiled baking pan and bake for one hour at 340°F.

Blueberry Muffins

3 cups carrot pulp

1 cup pineapple pulp

1 cup cold-pressed sesame oil or extra-virgin olive oil

3 eggs

1 cup honey

3 cups whole-grain flour

1 tbsp baking soda

1 tsp nutmeg

1 tbsp vanilla

1 cup fresh or frozen whole blueberries

Mix the carrots and the pineapple together; add the honey, eggs, vanilla and oil and mix. Sift together the dry ingredients and add to the mixture. Add the blueberries and stir in gently. Pour into muffin papers or greased muffin tins. Bake for 45 minutes at 350°F.

Pulp Sorbet

Take the pulp from any sweet fruit—peaches, apples, cherries, pears, apricots, pineapple, raspberries or strawberries. Collect the fruit until you have about three cups of pulp. Freeze in an ice-cube tray, and when frozen, put into a food processor with four ripe bananas and blend to the consistency of sorbet. Serve immediately.

Fruit Sauce

Take 1 cup of pulp from any sweet fruit, blend together with 2 tbsp honey or organic maple syrup and serve on toast or pancakes or over ice cream.

Total Juicing

Conventional juicers, whether they're centrifugal juicers or extruding juicers, all separate the juice from the pulp. You then have the option of using the pulp (which is what we strongly recommend since it is full of vitamins and minerals) or throwing it away. However, there is a whole new approach to juicing which is worth getting into. It is called total juicing or molecular juicing, and it requires a totally different piece of equipment than you use for ordinary juice making. This is a juicer that is ultrapowerful (see Resources).

Total juicing is a way of juicing the entire vegetable or fruit, from which you discard nothing. It is called molecular because it actually pulverizes the fruit or vegetable to such a fine degree that you are able to absorb the nutrients almost immediately. This form of juicing is wonderful for anyone who has a digestive problem, for babies, for anyone who wants to get large quantities of fiber (such as someone who is trying to lose weight) and for anyone whose digestion is less than perfect. It requires a very different approach than making the juices that we have looked at so far.

First of all, you need a very strong machine. Most ordinary blenders are not capable of molecular juicing. They will give you a mush that is highly unpleasant. Second, you need to remember that molecular juicing takes a lot more skill in what you mix with what, as if you mix combinations of fruits and vegetables together indiscriminately you can end up with a mess that tastes disgusting.

Molecular juicing is also a wonderful way of increasing the fiber in your diet. What is interesting is how many important ingredients in a fruit or vegetable are actually left in the fiber (another reason we urge you strongly not to discard your fiber). For instance, when you extract the juice from an orange, you get approximately 30IU of beta carotene, however 30IU more are discarded in the pulp. When you take similar measurements with a carrot, you get 14,000IU of carotene in the juice but another 9800IU remain in the fiber. With molecular juicing you get them all.

The juice you produce by placing your fruits or vegetables cut into convenient-sized pieces into a molecular juicer is not as sweet as that which is extracted from one of the more conventional juicers. This can be a good thing for people with blood sugar problems, since occasionally someone will find that the sweetness of carrot and apple, for instance, is such that it stimulates the pancreas to produce too much insulin. Generally speaking, however, this is not a problem, but any possibility of the problem can be completely eliminated by total juicing.

Total juices have a thicker texture, a totally different feeling in the mouth from that of the thin juices that come out of ordinary juice extractors. It is more like a nectar or a fruit smoothie that you get out of total juicing. Occasionally you might find you want to add a little sweetener in the form of maple syrup or natural, un-heated honey to your molecular juices. You will also need to add a little water or some ice cubes, generally speaking, in order to give a little more liquid for the pulverizing process to take place properly.

Soups & Sprouts

Another great thing to do if you have a blender capable of molecular juicing is to make your vegetable or fruit juice and then use it as an additive in your molecular juicing. For example, if you have made some carrot juice, use the juice as a base for making beautiful vegetable soups so you don't need to replace the water. It produces an absolutely delicious dish. Similarly, you can use your fruit juices as a base for making fruit frappes by mixing together the whole fruits—peaches, apricots and berries—in the blender with the juice that you have made from your conventional juicer.

Molecular juicing is a great way of using your sprouted alfalfa and mung beans. You simply take any vegetable or fruit juice, pour it into your blender and add a handful of your sprouts. Blend and drink immediately. The fiber in sprouted seeds is wonderful and it's a great way of getting the very best of both ways of juicing.

A blender capable of molecular juicing is an ideal way of making green drinks. After preparing a vegetable or fruit juice in an ordinary juicer, pour into the blender and add your green supplements, whether they come in the form of fresh green beet leaves, kale, spinach, or dandelion, then pour the juice made from the conventional juicer over the leaves and blend quickly and serve. You can also use the same method to add powdered wheat or barley grass to fresh juices. We try to use organic fruits and vegetables for molecular juicing just to be sure that we are protected from any intake of pesticides or herbicides. Here are some of our favorite recipes.

Fruit Medley

1/4 small pineapple, peeled and cut into spears
1 small orange, peeled but with the pith left on
1/2 apple
1/2 banana
1 tbsp maple syrup or honey

Cut all the fruit into bite-sized pieces, place in the blender with a few ice cubes and turn on at high speed for half a minute. Serve immediately.

Fruit Frappe

This is a lovely drink much like a frozen Daiquiri. Whether or not you add alcohol to it is up to you.

1 mango
1/2 banana
1/2 orange, peeled but with the pith left on
1 mango, peeled, with the inner peel removed

1/2 cup frozen strawberries
1/2 cup soymilk or low-fat yogurt
handful ice cubes

Cut the fruit into easy-to-manage pieces, toss into the
blender with the ice cubes and blend for 30 seconds at
high speed. Serve immediately.

Citrus Carrot Special

*This is a beautiful drink made even better if you chill all of
the ingredients before you use them.*

2 carrots
1/2 small pineapple
1 small orange

Peel the orange and pineapple and cut into bite-sized
pieces. Toss into the blender with a handful of ice cubes.
Blend and serve immediately.

Gazpacho

*You can also make wonderful raw soups as well as
uncooked warm soups using molecular juicing methods.*

2 cups spring water
1 medium-sized carrot
1 stick celery
2 green onions
4 ripe tomatoes, chilled
1 tsp vegetable bouillon powder
dash of white wine
1 tsp parsley

Place all the ingredients into the blender. Add two or
three ice cubes, blend for 30 seconds, sprinkle with
parsley and serve.

The High Life Diet: A 10-Day Program

Now let's see what High Life looks like. Here are the basic guidelines for ten days to reorient your eating habits permanently.

- Have juice for breakfast plus a green supplement either on its own or together with some fruit.
- Remember to chew your juices and drink your food. In other words sip your juices slowly so they have a chance to mix with the saliva in the mouth to get the full benefit of everything that is in them, and chew your foods until they turn into liquids.
- Avoid eating between meals since this slows down the stomach's emptying and encourages food still in the stomach to ferment; it also creates false appetite. If you are hungry, have a glass of fresh juice or lots of spring water between meals.
- Try to leave four to five hours between meals. This is the time your body needs to efficiently and completely digest its previous meal.
- Make mealtimes a pleasure
- Eat slowly and chew thoroughly. Not only does this increase the enjoyment of your food it also means that you digest your food properly so you don't end up with digestive disturbances.
- Drink as much water as you like, virtually the more the better. But don't drink water with meals—give yourself twenty minutes water-free before a meal and half an hour afterwards.
- Try to take your main meal at lunch and the light meal in the evening. This is an ideal way to live since you sleep much deeper and better if you don't eat heavily at night. However, you must suit your

eating to your lifestyle and when you have to have a main meal at night, enjoy it.

A DAY ON THE HIGH LIFE DIET

Begin the day with a cup of hot or cold spring water with the juice of half a lemon and a little honey or organic maple syrup if desired.

Throughout the day drink as much spring water as you like. If you are hungry between meals have another glass of juice, preferably green.

SALADS

Trio Salads

Trio Salads are best of all. The principles of making them are simple. Mix together three vegetables—one root, one bulb (or "fruit") vegetable and one leaf vegetable. Garnish with fresh or dried herbs and add dressing.

Root Vegetables: carrots, celery root, turnips, onions, leeks, beet, radishes, white radishes, etc.

Bulb or "fruit" vegetables: tomatoes, red and green peppers, fennel, avocado, cucumber, cauliflower, celery, broccoli, zucchini, mushrooms, etc.

Leaf vegetables: lettuce, young dandelion leaves, young beet tops, red or white cabbage, Brussels sprouts, spring onions, spring greens, spinach, chicory, endive, etc. Watercress, cress and sprouted grains and seeds can be used in any combination or on their own or as a garnish.

To increase a salad's protein content you can sprinkle it with the three-seed mixture, or mixed nuts or sprouted seeds or grains, or add some soft goat cheese, free-range chicken, chopped hard-boiled eggs, prawns, etc.

Sprout Salad

Mix two or three kinds of sprouted grains or seeds (a handful of each) in a bowl, add half a sliced avocado and season with fresh basil and chives. Garnish with black olives and dress with garlic dressing.

Spinach Splendor

2 cups spinach
1 cup fresh mushrooms

Remove stems and veins of spinach. Slice mushrooms finely and mix together. Toss in garlic dressing and sprinkle with basil or sunflower seeds.

Red Slaw

1 cups grated cabbage
1 grated carrot
grated green pepper
1 tbsp honey
a pinch of celery seeds

Toss with salad dressing and serve.

Sunshine Salad

The fresh pineapple gives this salad a tropical taste. Make sure your pineapple is ripe by pulling out one of its center leaves; if it comes out easily it is ready to eat.

1 fresh pineapple
2 carrots
2 sticks celery
1/2 green pepper
a few crisp lettuce leaves
2 handfuls raisins

BREAKFAST	MAIN MEAL	LIGHT MEAL
Large glass fresh raw fruit juice—apple, orange, grape, grapefruit, etc., or a recipe of your choice. To this add either some green leaves such as dandelion, beet, spinach, the juice from one of the cereal grasses, or a teaspoon to a tablespoon of one of the cereal grass supplements, such as green barley, stirred into your glass of juice. You can drink as much more juice as you like (with or without the extra green) and you can also have a piece of fruit or a bunch of grapes and as much herbal tea as you like, sweetened with a little honey or maple syrup.	If at all possible, make this meal at lunchtime since you will digest your food better and sleep better if you eat light in the evening.	Glass of fresh vegetable or fruit juice
		A salad or light soup
	Large glass of fresh, raw vegetable juice; choose any mixture you like—carrot, raw beet, celery, cucumber, cabbage, tomato, spinach, etc.—or one of the recipes at the end of the book.	Several slices of whole-grain bread or a bowl of granola
		Herbal tea or coffee substitute
	A big salad—one of the best of all are the Trio Salads (see below) together with some grilled fish, lambs' liver, free-range chicken, game, a tofu dish or an omelette	
	Steamed or wok-fried vegetables	
	Herb tea or coffee substitute	

1/2 tsp celery seeds

1 tsp dry mustard mixed with vinaigrette

Wash and crisp the lettuce leaves in the fridge. Peel the pineapple (it is not necessary to core it) and cut it into fairly small cubes. Coarsely grate the carrots, and finely chop the celery and green pepper, and add them to the pineapple cubes. Add the raisins, soaked in water for a few hours to plump them up. Sprinkle with celery seeds and serve on a bed of crisp lettuce leaves. Serve with a spicy, mustardy mayonnaise or French dressing.

Orange Orange Salad

A surprising combination... but it works!

4 carrots

1–2 cups white cabbage

6 oranges

2 handfuls raisins or small seedless grapes

4 tsp sesame seeds

Coarsely chop the carrots. Juice four of the oranges and blend the juice with the carrots until you have a smooth mixture. Finely shred or grate the cabbage and put it in a bowl with the raisins or grapes. Pour the carrot mixture over it and lightly mix with a fork. Sprinkle with the sesame seeds and garnish with the two remaining oranges, peeled and sliced.

Summer Symphony

This salad is an exciting play of colors and shapes—the more variety the better.

1 bunch lettuce

1 cup small cauliflower florets

2 celery stalks (finely chopped)

2 carrots (finely grated or cut into matchsticks)
6 cherry tomatoes
4 radishes (sliced)
1 green pepper (cut into thin strips)
watercress
fresh sweet corn or alfalfa sprouts to garnish

Place the lettuce leaves, torn into bite size pieces or shredded, into a bowl—a clear glass bowl is nice for this one so that all the beautiful colors show through it. Prepare the vegetables and arrange in layers in the bowl, keeping the watercress for decoration. Dress with a thinned mayonnaise dressing, perhaps blended with a tomato or two, and top with sweet corn or alfalfa sprouts, and sprigs of watercress.

Sprout Magic Salad

Make a base with alfalfa or mung sprouts and around the dish arrange:

grated carrot
red cabbage
white cabbage
beet
sliced mushrooms
black olives
green onions

Sprinkle raisins over the grated vegetables and spoon over a rich dressing.

SALAD DRESSINGS

Basic Dressing

Mix one part lemon juice and two parts extra-virgin olive oil or four parts mashed avocado. Add herbs, garlic, mustard or honey to this base.

Tomato Dressing

3–5 tomatoes
2 tbsp lemon juice
1/2 tsp basil

Put into a blender and liquefy. Store in the fridge.

Avocado-Tomato Dressing

4 small tomatoes
1 avocado
2 tbsp lemon juice
dash of Tabasco
crushed clove of garlic or dash of garlic powder

Mix in blender. Store in the fridge.

Yogurt & Egg Dressing

1 egg yolk
1½ cups nonfat yogurt or tofu
3 tbsp lemon juice or cider vinegar
pinch cayenne pepper
fresh or dried herbs to taste
2 tsp honey

Put ingredients into the top of a double boiler and stir over hot water until the mixture thickens. Refrigerate to serve cold or use hot on hot potato salad or hot rice salad.

Thousand Island Dressing

1 hard-boiled egg, chopped
5 tsp celery, finely chopped
3 tbsp onion, finely chopped
2 tbsp black olives, chopped
1 tbsp green pepper, finely chopped
1/2 cup nonfat yogurt

Mix all ingredients and serve chilled

Non-Oil Vinaigrette

3 tbsp dried nonfat milk
1/2 tsp Dijon mustard
2 tsp honey
dash of pepper
pinch of basil
1 clove garlic, crushed
2 tbsp vinegar

Mix ingredients, adding vinegar last. Beat well or blend until smooth. Chill and use the same day.

RAW SOUPS

Cucumber

1 cup low-fat yogurt or soymilk
1/2 cucumber, peeled and sliced
sprig of mint
1 tsp lemon juice

Blend and serve sprinkled with parsley.

Gazpacho

4–6 peeled tomatoes
3 carrots

2 sticks of celery
dash of cayenne

Put through a juicer. Sprinkle with chopped chives and
diced green pepper.

Avocado Smoothie

3/4 cup low-fat yogurt or tofu
1/2 avocado
1/4 diced red pepper
1 tsp lemon juice
1 chopped green onion
dash of Tabasco

Blend and serve.

Carrot Chowder

1 cup nuts (almonds, hazels or pecans)
1 cup low-fat yogurt
2 egg yolks
small clove of garlic, pressed
juice of two lemons
1 tbsp olive oil
2 tsp vegetable bouillon powder
3 cups carrot juice (using about 12 big carrots)
ice cubes
1/2 green pepper
2 green onions
chopped parsley

Grind the nuts finely and blend them with the yogurt,
egg yolks, pressed garlic, lemon juice, olive oil and
seasoning. Juice the carrots into a jar with ice cubes in it,
then slowly add the juice and ice to the yogurt mixture,

stirring well. Serve sprinkled with a mixture of finely chopped green pepper, green onion and parsley.

Flamingo Soup

2 medium-sized beets
10 carrots
1 small head celery
ice
juice of one lemon
4–6 tomatoes
2 handfuls almonds
1 tbsp fresh thyme
1 tbsp fresh basil
vegetable bouillon powder to taste
6 tbsp yogurt
chives

Juice the beets, carrots and celery and put into an airtight jar with some ice and the lemon juice. Blend the tomatoes, almonds, thyme, basil and bouillon powder. Combine the two mixtures and serve in bowls with a spoonful of yogurt and a sprinkling of chopped chives.

Fresh Green Soup

2 avocados, peeled and stoned
3 cups apple juice
juice of 1/2 lemon
parsley
2 tsp tamari
1 tsp vegetable bouillon powder
ground ginger
1 zucchini
1 stick celery

handful of alfalfa and mung sprouts
sliced mushrooms or slivered almonds

Combine the avocados, apple juice, lemon juice, parsley, tamari, vegetable bouillon and a pinch of ginger in the blender. Grate the zucchini and finely dice the celery and mix them with the sprouts. Now pour on the avocado sauce. Serve sprinkled with sliced mushroom or flakes of almond.

MUESLI

Live Muesli

1–2 tbsp breakfast oats, soaked overnight in a little spring
  water
1 grated apple (or mango, peach, strawberries, etc.)
1/2 cup low-fat yogurt

Mix all the ingredients and sprinkle with toasted seeds or mixed nuts.

7

PARTY TIME

Raw juices are seriously good for you. But who wants to be serious all the time? Not only is it OK to have fun, but making time to relax and enjoy yourself is crucial. Raw juices are not just for the abstemious and self-consciously healthy; they're also utterly delicious and appeal to the hedonist inside all of us. This chapter is dedicated to the pursuit of pleasure.

Naturally sweet, fruity drinks are the healthy alternative to the sugary soda that usually fuels children's parties and tends to make kids hyperactive. We can't guarantee that your child's birthday party won't end in tears if you give the young guests raw juice instead of carbonated drinks and fruit smoothies instead of ice cream sundaes, but our experience suggests that children will get a lot less fractious and play more happily together if you do.

Not that there is anything childish about the kind of fruit punches suggested later in this chapter. Mixed with alcohol, freshly extracted juices make the most seductive cocktails and are guaranteed to make any social gathering flow easily. Obviously, getting intoxicated on a regular basis is not a great idea, but it's arguable that the expansive conviviality induced by alcohol helps us all to remember that we're only human.

Raw juices make the most sublime mixers for alcohol, but at any adult gathering there will be a proportion of people who do not wish to drink alcohol. Raw juice is a great leveler at parties because you can devise cocktails that taste just as good with or without a shot of alcohol. Teetotalers and hard-core hedonists can then mingle with impunity, all cradling glasses that look the same.

The first time we observed this phenomenon was at a marathon poetry performance for which we concocted a Purple Poetry Potion. It being an evening of beat poetry reading, we used beet juice, mixed with apple and pear, with or without vodka. Beat poets have various needs. Some wanted a stiff drink to steady their nerves; others were in rehab and scrupulously avoided stiff drinks. All, however, were intrigued by the profoundly earthy potion and some were moved to new heights of lyricism.

Smoothies

Children of all ages love smoothies, made in a blender (see Resources) rather than a juicer, which is particularly appropriate for liquefying bananas. Bananas are not totally unjuiceable if you use very soft specimens and follow them through your juicer with very watery fruits such as melons, which will help to wash the thick banana through the machine. However, using a blender to make banana drinks is a lot easier and less wasteful.

Many soft, exotic fruits including peaches, mangoes, papaya and pineapple work well in the blender (so long as you take care to remove all their skin and pits). Smoothies are especially good when blended with plain yogurt, which give them the texture of milkshakes, or melted ice cream with a low fat content. Use low-fat yogurt, or Greek yogurt made with goat milk. These are a few of our favorite combinations:

Banana & Pineapple Smoothie

1 banana
2 spears pineapple
3 tbsp low-fat yogurt

Peel the banana and break into chunks. Remove the fibrous skin from the pineapple and cut into spears, then into chunks. Put all the ingredients into the blender and blend until smooth.

Mango & Peach Smoothie

If you have problem getting the stone out of a mango, the trick is to use a tablespoon. Cut around the edge of the fruit with a sharp knife. Slide the spoon over one side of the stone and twist it.

1 mango
3 peaches
3 tbsp low-fat yogurt

Remove the stones from the peaches and the mango and cut both fruits into chunks. Put all the ingredients into the blender and blend until smooth.

Banana & Peach Smoothie with Strawberries

1 banana
1 peach
12 strawberries

3 tbsp low-fat yogurt

Peel the banana and break it up into chunks. Remove the pit from the peach and chop the fruit into chunks. Remove the green stems from the strawberries. Put all the ingredients into the blender and blend until smooth.

Cantaloupe & Papaya Smoothie

Cantaloupes, with their rough skins and flesh of a delicate pink, orange or green color, produce a rich, sweet juice that blends well with other exotic fruits.

1/2 cantaloupe

1 papaya

Cut the melon into spears; remove the flesh from the skin. Peel the papaya and scrape out the seeds. Chop both fruits into chunks, put into the blender and blend until smooth. You can substitute mango for the papaya and you may also like to add a piece of citrus fruit—an orange, or maybe a lime—to add another dimension.

Banana & Honeydew with Apricot

A mild nectar that is quite thick and is best served over ice, or thinned with a splash of spring water. Less than half a honeydew should be more than adequate..

1 banana

1/3 honeydew melon

6 apricots

Peel the banana, remove the pits from the apricots and cut the melon into spears, then slice the flesh into chunks and remove from the skin. Put all the ingredients into a blender and blend until smooth.

Exotic Fruit Cocktails

International commerce has blurred the seasons so that there is an abundant supply of exotic fruits in the supermarkets all year round, but summer is the right time to make the most of them. Exotic, fruity cocktails made with a centrifugal juice extractor have an amazingly creamy texture and are perfect refreshments for a hot afternoon. For garden parties and barbecues, they're ideal.

Later we'll explore the alcohol connection, but in the meantime it might occur to you that the recipe suggestions below could be enlivened with the addition of a jigger of rum, or maybe a splash of vodka. Far be it for us to discourage experimentation. On a practical note, the ideal way to chill these drinks is with a handful of crushed ice in the bottom of each glass, but it's also a good idea to keep all the ingredients refrigerated or iced in an insulated box.

Melon Medley with Berries

You can mix different kinds of melon juice together to create sublime blends, such as Honeyloupe (Cantaloupe and Honeydew, which is even better with a hint of ginger). Add summer berries to perk up their flavor. Use this recipe as the basis for experimentation:

1 slice honeydew
1 slice watermelon
12 raspberries

Peel the waxy outer skin from the honeydew and wash the rind of the watermelon. Juice the ingredients together and serve over ice.

Cantaloupe & Carrot with a Twist of Lemon

An intriguing and refreshing combination with a marvelous color.

1/2 cantaloupe melon
1/2 lemon
3 carrots

Remove the rind from the melon with a vegetable peeler and remove the skin from the lemon, leaving the pith. Juice together with the carrots, leaving one of the carrots to put through your juicer last.

Kiwi & Grape with Honeydew

Kiwis do not have to be peeled before juicing, so long as they're thoroughly washed. They have a slightly sharp flavor that blends well with melon, and this juice is light, green and refreshing.

1/4 honeydew melon
2 kiwifruits
12 green grapes

Peel the waxy rind from the melon and put through the juicer with the other ingredients.

Orangeade

Forget about proprietary canned drinks and make your own sparkling summer cooler.

2 oranges
1/4 lemon
1/4 lime
Soda or sparkling spring water

Peel the citrus fruits, leaving on the white pith, and serve, topping up the glass with soda or sparkling water.

Orange & Raspberry

A terrific, summery combination with an amazing color.

2 oranges
handful raspberries (about 12)

Peel the oranges, leaving on the pith, and juice as usual with the raspberries.

Pineapple & Orange

Pineorange is a great, refreshing combination. Oranges vary considerably in juiciness; you'll need one big, firm and luscious orange or two smaller specimens.

2 spears pineapple (about 1/2 a smallish fruit)
1 or 2 oranges

Peel the fibrous outer skin from the pineapple and the waxy skin from the orange, leaving the pith. Juice together.

The Alcohol Connection

The juices used in most cocktail bars come out of a carton and are rarely fresh, but you can set up a raw juice bar to make drinks that taste superb and are nourishing as well as intoxicating! Raw juice is especially useful for mixing with clear spirits, particularly vodka, but be careful how much you add, since raw juice cocktails are deceptively easy to drink. Remember the golden rule of moderation in all things.

Cocktails were originally invented during prohibition to disguise the harsh taste of illegally distilled hooch.

However, we never touch cheap liquor and recommend that you stick to the more refined premium brands, which have been distilled to a higher specification and will leave you with less of a hangover.

The exception to the quality rule is when mixing juices with sparkling wine to make the ultimate party punch. Using real Champagne is an unnecessary extravagance when there is now such a variety of good, cheap sparkling wines from Spain and the New World on the market. Here are a few of our favorite sparklers:

Mimosa/Bellini/Titiani

Mimosa, or Buck's Fizz, is a simple half-and-half mixture of Champagne and orange juice. The same drink made with peaches, or apricots is a Bellini; one made with red grapes is a Titiani. A tip is to add the juice to the sparkling wine, which will reduce the over-frothing that tends to happen if you try it the other way round.

Champagne Cooler

1/2 a small pineapple
1 lemon
sparkling wine

Fill half a tall glass with ice. Juice the fruit and pour it over the ice, then top with sparkling wine.

Mango/Papaya Go-Go

Use either mango or papaya to make this unusual and startlingly good party fuel.

1 large, ripe mango or papaya
2 kiwifruits
1 big carrot

Sparkling wine

Remove the flesh from the mango, or peel and remove the seeds from the papaya. Juice with the kiwifruit and the carrot. Pour into a glass, stir and top with sparkling wine.

Sangria Real

Possibly the most popular summer party drink, Sangria, made with freshly extracted fruit juices mixed with red wine and given a sparkle with a splash of soda is an unbeatable way to relax on a hot day.

Red wine
1 orange
1/4 lemon
1/2 lime
Soda or sparkling spring water

Fill half a tall glass with ice and pour in a wineglass measure of red wine. Remember to leave the pith on the citrus fruits, juice them and pour over the red wine and enough soda or sparkling mineral water to fill the glass. Stir and drink through a straw.

MARGARITA TIME

Distilled from the fermented juice of an Agave cactus, tequila is most often drunk in the form of a margarita. The classic margarita is made with lime juice and Cointreau and served in a salt-rimmed glass, but frozen margaritas, like alcoholic slush puppies, have become ubiquitous. If you have a masticating juicer, like the Champion, you can make excellent frozen Margaritas simply by freezing the fruit before you put it through the juicer. If using a centrifugal extractor, freezing the fruit will reduce its juice yield, but will chill the drink.

Strawberry Margarita

If you can find a blood orange to make your margarita, so much the better.

2 oz. tequila
12 frozen strawberries
1 orange
1/2 lime

Measure the tequila into a glass. Juice the fruit in the order listed and pour over the tequila. Serve.

RUM-BASED DRINKS

Rum, made from molasses, is ideally suited to mixing with fruit juices. Bacardi—a blend of white rums from different countries—is the single biggest alcohol brand in the world, but many tropical islands produce their own brands of rum and each has its own characteristics although some, such as Wray & Nephew's overproof white rum, are pretty hard to take unless heavily diluted. Feel free to experiment with darker rums like Myers, Cockspur and even Bacardi Gold.

Piña Colada

The classic tropical cocktail. You can buy coconut cream in cans or, as a last resort, use one of the proprietary brands like Malibu, which is ready-mixed with rum.

2 spears of pineapple
3 large tbsp coconut cream
2 oz. white rum
a maraschino cherry

Serve over crushed ice, garnished with a maraschino cherry on top.

Rum Punch

Not a Planters' Punch, which is made with simple syrup and flavored with lime and Angostura, but a long and exotic, slightly fizzy drink. Use the biggest, ripest mangoes you can lay your hands on.

1 mango
1/2 lemon
1 lime
2 oz. dark rum
soda water

Juice the mango and the citrus fruits, leaving on the white pith. Put some crushed ice into a glass and pour the rum over it. Pour in the fruit juices, stir and top with a splash of soda.

Euphoria

Curaçao is a West Indian liquor made from bitter oranges (originally from the island of Curaçao) which is now available in a range of colors. The original remains best for this recipe.

2 oz. white rum
1/2 oz. curaçao
1/2 pink grapefruit
1 spear pineapple

Measure the alcohol into a glass half-filled with crushed ice. Juice the grapefruit and pineapple and stir into the rum. The curaçao can be floated on top of the drink or stirred into it.

VODKA-BASED DRINKS

Vodka is increasingly popular, particularly with people who don't like the taste of alcohol, because it has little or no flavor and can easily be disguised by mixing with fruit juices. We prefer to use a premium brand, such as Absolut, which is exceptionally pure and won't give you a hangover. When traveling, seek out the extra-strength, red label Absolut in duty-free stores.

Harvey Wallbanger

A screwdriver, vodka mixed with orange juice, is the most basic vodka cocktail, and this is a more sophisticated variation, with the addition of a spoonful of Galliano, the spicy, herby Italian liquor sold in tall bottles, floated on top.

2 oz. vodka
1 large, ripe orange
1 tbsp of Galliano

Measure the vodka into a glass, over ice. Juice the orange and mix it in. Gently float the Galliano on top.

Lucky Jim

A longer version of this classic variation of the Dry Martini, this recipe makes a light green and deceptively refreshing cocktail. A great aperitif, this recipe also works well with gin.

2 oz. vodka
1¼-inch section of cucumber
1 stalk of celery
a splash of dry vermouth (such as Noilly Prat)

Put some ice cubes in the bottom of a tall glass and add a splash of vodka. Leave to stand while juicing the cucumber and celery. Add the juice and the vodka, stir and serve with a stalk of parsley to garnish.

Ultimate Bloody Mary

There must be more bloody mary recipes than for any other mixed drink, but most are predicated on canned tomato juice and require wakening-up with a dash of sherry and a range of garnishes. This one uses raw juice and doesn't require such extraneous adornments, unless you are partial to them.

2 oz. vodka
3 ripe tomatoes
1 stalk celery
2-inch section of cucumber
a dash of Tabasco, or Worcestershire Sauce
salt and cayenne pepper or grated horseradish

Measure the vodka over ice. Juice the remaining ingredients, stir and serve with your choice of seasonings.

8

QUICK FIX

Because raw juice is the richest available source of vitamins, minerals and enzymes, it is the best possible tonic for promoting all-around health and general well-being. Most people who embrace the Juice High lifestyle find that the minor complaints that used to irritate them fade away as the body rebalances itself, and they become accustomed to feeling perfectly fine, all of the time. The key to building and sustaining an indomitable physiology, one in which the body is strong, focused and invulnerable to illness, is the consumption of the broadest possible range of juices. However, each juice has specific therapeutic properties and this chapter shows how you can use raw juice to treat a range of common complaints.

Modern medical science tends to have a nuts-and-bolts approach in prescribing drugs to treat the symptoms of illness, frequently without paying attention to the underlying causes of the condition. Natural health practitioners try to take a holistic view, seeing the body as a complete organism with many parts, all of which must operate synergistically for the whole being to be healthy.

Illness is the result of disharmony, or a chemical imbalance in the body caused by nutritional deficiency. Most of the conditions described below will respond rapidly when you drink the recommended juices, but do remember that they are only recommendations, not prescriptions.

Any attempt to treat a medical condition should always come under the direction of a competent physician. We are only reporters, albeit with a profound interest in helping ourselves and others to maximize our potential for positive health, which includes being able to live at a high level of energy, intelligence and creativity. For all three are expressions of harmony within a living, organic system.

ACNE

A lot of acne is the result of eating a diet high in sugar and low in fiber. When the body is not eliminating waste properly, the pores of the skin become blocked. It is very important to make sure that you eat plenty of vegetables that are rich in fiber (not wheat or wheat bran, as in wholegrain bread, as this tends to clog up a lot of people who suffer from acne and skin problems). Steer clear of processed convenience foods full of the kind of hydrogenated fats you find in margarines, and stick to using olive oil for your salads and wok frying. Do a detox and use the High Life Diet, emphasizing the fresh vegetables and fruits. Avoid dairy products and any kind of junk food.

Carrot juice is very beneficial for acne, but the green juices are supreme. Drink lots and lots of fresh carrot juice, to which you add as much green as you can manage as often as you can manage it. The best sources of green lightning are cabbage and kale, beet and turnip tops, watercress and spinach, and parsley and dandelion leaves.

Recipes that can help with acne problems include:

- Ginger Spice
- Green Friend
- Carrot High
- Chlorophyll Plus
- Carrot & Apple

ALLERGIES

It can be enormously frustrating to suffer these unpleasant reactions to substances that other people seem to cope with so easily, mostly because they tend to be treated as though they have a single cause. All allergies, from the classic antibody-antigen reactions that cause the release of histamine, to food allergies, which can act quite differently, must be treated holistically. That means supported by diet, rest, stress management and the elimination of any possible trigger foods or environmental chemicals.

Sugar is the first thing that needs to be eliminated completely from the diet. Cut out packaged convenience foods that are full of additives such as aspartame—the sulphites in prepared meat foods—and monosodium glutamate (MSG). Many allergic people have an overgrowth of Candida albicans yeast in their bodies and need to address this at the same time. Milk products are best avoided by anyone with any sort of allergic condition.

Most allergic reactions occur when the body is over-acidic. A highly alkaline diet, such as a Raw Energy-type diet, plus lots of alfalfa sprouts or juice, which are rich in mineral salts, can help tremendously to create the right internal environment and help you to become allergy-free. Celery is also good. Grapefruit, orange, cantaloupe and parsley are rich in the bioflavonoids; spinach, kale and sweet peppers are rich in B6, which can be particularly helpful for many sensitivities; garlic, spinach and cauliflower are a good source of molybdenum, a trace element that tends to be deficient in people who are sensitive to the sulphites and MSG.

Recipes that can help with allergy problems include:
- Red Cool
- Celery Sticks
- Parsley Passion
- Sprout Special

ANEMIA

Anemia occurs either when there is a decrease in the total number of red blood cells, or in the volume of the blood, or when red blood cells become abnormal in shape or size. This condition tends to make you pale, weak and inhibits your resistance to infection. It often creates insomnia, leading to irritability and depression and causing chronic fatigue. There are a number of different underlying deficiencies that are present when one is anemic, of which iron is important in order to be able to form new red blood cells, but so too are folic acid and vitamin B12 in helping to rebuild red blood cells. If anemia persists, consult your doctor because it could possibly be the result of abnormalities in the production of hemoglobin itself.

Green drinks and green foods are essential for anemia. They are rich in folic acid and many of them are rich in iron, particularly watercress, spinach, beet tops, dandelion leaves and the brassicas. Vegetables that are particularly beneficial include parsley, green pepper, beet tops, carrot, kale, spinach and asparagus. Berries can be very useful, particularly for women (and are similarly good for menstrual cramps, morning sickness and calming labor pains, not to mention sea sickness, yeast infections and poor circulation).

Try to drink as many green drinks as possible. To each glass add a teaspoon of spirulina, which is extremely rich in B12, and shake or blend well.

Recipes that can help with anemia include:
- Green Zinger
- Dandelion Plus
- Red Flag
- Beet Treat
- Easy Does It
- Double Whammy

ARTHRITIS

Both osteoarthritis and rheumatoid arthritis have been successfully treated with juice therapy, which is particularly beneficial if the patient has not been on long-term drug treatment. Osteoarthritis affects the bones and joints with symptoms such as swelling of soft tissues, local tenderness, restricted movement, bony swellings and crackings of the joints as well as stiffness after resting. The more the joint is used in osteoarthritis, the worse the pain generally becomes. Rheumatoid arthritis produces inflammatory conditions in the joints and the structures surrounding joints, as well as a feeling of weakness, often low-grade fever, long-term fatigue, pain and stiffness. Rheumatoid arthritis is increasingly considered an autoimmune reaction where the body has actually developed antibodies against its own tissues.

In both rheumatoid and osteoarthritis, certain things are essential. First, that you cut out foods from the nightshade family such as potatoes, eggplant, tomatoes, and peppers. Secondly, in the case of osteoarthritis, that you avoid citrus fruits such as limes, lemons, oranges and grapefruits. In the tradition of natural medicine, they are believed to contribute to the inflammation.

With both forms of arthritis, it is important to avoid all convenience foods and refined foods such as white sugar, white flour, processed foods that contain chemical additives, and alcohol. Consider the possibility that you might have some sort of a sensitivity or allergic reaction to food, perhaps to wheat or to dairy products. Try eliminating wheat flour and everything made from it, as well as all dairy products from your diet for three weeks and see if it makes a significant difference. In the case of rheumatoid arthritis, it can be useful (if you are not a vegetarian) to eat more cold-water fish, such as tuna, sardines, salmon and mackerel, all of which contain the essential fatty acid known as omega 3. Many people with arthritis fair better on a low-fat vegetarian diet.

Vegetables to incorporate into your juices include carrot, beet tops, broccoli, turnip, grapes, kale, cabbage, all dark green vegetables, apple and ginger. Pineapple is particularly good for rheumatoid arthritis since it contains the enzyme bromelin, which has anti-inflammatory properties.

Dandelion juice is excellent, especially for rheumatoid arthritis. Pick the dandelion greens carefully, from places which have are not likely to have been sprayed and are not along the verges of roads where they may have picked up heavy metals such as lead from air pollution. Cut off the leaves and wash then well before putting them through the juicer. If you are used to drinking green juices, you can actually drink dandelion juice on its own, or mixed equally with carrot. It also mixes well with a little watercress. If you are not used to drinking green juices, it can be useful to start with a delicious sweet juice such as carrot and apple and then gradually increase the levels of dandelion you are putting into it. Dandelion also has the ability to create an amazing high once the juice is assimilated into the liver, which usually takes about half an hour. But go easy, for if your digestive system is not used to green juices this can be too much of a shock. Start with small amounts and increase gradually.

Recipes that can help with arthritis include:
- Pineapple Green
- Green Goddess
- Green Wow
- Sprouting o' the Green
- Top of the Beet
- Popeye Punch
- Pineapple Special
- Pineapple Green
- Ginger Berry
- Red Genius

ASTHMA

The theory is that asthma comes in two forms. One kind is said to be caused by specific allergens either in the air or food; the other is said to have no particular cause. Most experts in natural medicine, however, find that there is always an allergic element, as there is also always an emotional one in any kind of asthma or any other condition in which the symptoms include spasms of the bronchial tubes and swelling of the mucus membrane.

Perhaps the most important remedy is to eliminate from the diet any foods that create mucous in the body. This means not eating dairy products, coffee, tea, chocolate, wheat and convenience foods. Many asthmatics find they do best when they eliminate from their diet not only wheat but also other grains as well (except for buckwheat, which is not a true grain, and brown rice or millet). Asthmatics seem to be more affected by food allergies than other people, which can result in inflammation of the bronchial tubes that causes an even stronger reaction to pollen and air pollutants such as sulphur-dioxide and to smoke. Asthma also appears to weaken the adrenal glands, so handling it means living on a low-allergy diet in which at least 50 percent of the foods that you eat are taken raw.

Juices that are particularly rich in magnesium, which relaxes the bronchial muscle, are particularly useful, including: turnip, watercress, kale, turnip greens, parsley, collard greens, carrots, asparagus and beet tops. A couple of tablespoons of lemon juice added to any glass of fresh raw juice is a traditional treatment for asthma, as is molasses, which can be a useful "additive" to a glass of any juice. Other "additives" which are equally useful include fresh ginger, onions and garlic (in small quantities, if you wish to keep your friends).

Recipes that can help with asthma problems include:
- Carrot High
- Hi Mag
- Glorious Grapefruit
- Hi NRG
- Potassium Punch
- Leslie's Cocktail

CELLULITE

Orange-peel skin, the lumps and bumps that are so hard to get rid of, even in slim women, can be shed provided you take a total body approach to the issue. Women with cellulite are often constipated, even if they have one bowel movement a day, and they also tend to have poor lymphatic drainage, so that wastes are not eliminated properly. In addition, many women with cellulite suffer from poor liver function and an underactive thyroid.

Foods that are rich in bioflavonoids, such as sweet peppers, tomatoes, cabbage and parsley, citrus fruits (incorporate the pithy, white covering inside the peel in your juices), are important because the help strengthen the capillaries so you don't get leakage and the pockets of water that create *pea d'orange* flesh. Vitamin C is also important to strengthen the capillaries, as is zinc. If you want to shed cellulite permanently, shift the percentage of raw foods in your diet so that you are consuming between 50 and 75 percent of your foods raw. Use skin brushing, cut out *all* convenience foods, which are replete with junk fats and chemicals, and eliminate coffee and tea.

Remember that cellulite is slow to form and slow to clear, but it will go away provided you are persistent. These juices will be beneficial:

- Ginger Berry
- Hi Mag
- Ginger's Best
- Waterfall
- Potassium Power
- Pineapple Green

COLDS

The common cold has for generations been considered among natural health practitioners to be a means of the body eliminating waste when it has become overloaded. When you feel yourself coming down with a cold, eliminate all dairy products from your diet and all foods with sugar in them. Do a Juice Blitz and follow that by following The High Life Diet for at least for the next week or so.

Juicing for colds has two goals. The first is to strengthen the immune system and for this you need lots of green—kale, parsley, green pepper, watercress—which contain plenty of antioxidants such as beta carotene (don't forget your carrots too) as well as vitamin C, chlorophyll and all of those as yet unidentified plant factors which are so strengthening to the body. The second aspect of juicing for colds is in many ways the most important of all, which is elimination. This is using juices from vegetables and fruits that help eliminate waste from the system. Vegetables that are particularly good include: lemon, apricot, garlic, parsley, ginger, watercress, kale, radish, spinach, apple, pear and tomato.

Recipes that can help with colds include:
- Sweet and Spicy
- Salad Juice
- Pineapple Grapefruit Drink
- Hi Mag
- Carrot High
- Red Genius
- Ginger Spice
- Atomic Liftoff
- Beet, Carrot & Orange

CONSTIPATION

Constipation is the hidden condition that, according to natural health practitioners, is so widespread that it would be hard to quantify it. These experts insist that very few of us are actually cleansing our colon as thoroughly as we should. Most people find that when they begin to take juices and eat a higher percentage of their foods raw, their constipation clears by itself and they begin to have two or three bowel movements a day. It is essential to overall health that the bowels function really well, for if fecal matter stays in the colon, then harmful substances from the natural bacteria that live in the bowel can contribute to the development not only of many specific ailments such as hemorrhoids, varicose veins, hernias, cellulite, flatulence, obesity, insomnia, bad breath, indigestion, diverticulitis, but also to degenerative diseases from cancer to coronary heart disease, diabetes and even long-term depression.

One of the best natural remedies for constipation is rhubarb. Rhubarb is a vegetable but is usually thought of as a fruit. It is rich in calcium, phosphorus, iron, sodium, potassium, vitamin A, folic acid, vitamin C and magnesium. Raw rhubarb, like spinach, also contains oxalic acid, which you don't want to get too much of. Therefore, rhubarb is not an ingredient we would use daily in any of our juices. Rhubarb is also useful for intestinal parasites, for intestinal gas, and rhubarb juice applied externally is traditionally used to treat leg ulcers, bedsores and wounds. However, rhubarb juice and spinach juice should not be taken by anyone who suffers from kidney stones because of their high oxalic acid content.

Getting over constipation is usually a simple matter once you begin to juice, but there are a number of juices that are especially useful during the transition stage. Rhubarb, apples, spinach, prunes and pears all have a natural laxative effect.

Recipes that can help with constipation include:
• Rhubarb Radiance
• Spinapple
• Apple & Pear
• Ginger's Best
• Tropical Prune
• Sprout Special
• Black Watermelon

- Beet Treat
- Carrot, Beet, Celery & Tomato

DEPRESSION

Feeling depressed is not just a psychological condition. Very often that sense of purposelessness, emptiness, feelings of worthlessness and guilt come from a biochemical imbalance in the body. Internal pollution is a major cause, which is why a Juice Blitz plus a week on the High Life Diet shifts depression for many people.

Sugar and caffeine should be avoided, and it is important to check for any food allergies. Nobody who is depressed should be eating convenience foods, even those so-called comfort foods that are supposed to cheer us up. The neurotransmitters—hormones in the brain that control feeling—are derived from the food we eat, and in order for them to be proper brain chemicals, the food has got to be good. Serotonin is a particularly significant neurotransmitter that is derived from the amino acid tryptophan. When there are adequate levels of serotonin in the brain, the mood tends to be elevated and sleep patterns are normal. When they tumble, you get mood distortions and interrupted sleep patterns. A meal rich in complex carbohydrates helps the body absorb tryptophan and therefore supplies what is necessary for it to produce serotonin.

Bananas, figs and dates are rich in tryptophan. Carbohydrates in the form of a piece of toast and a banana before bed can help tremendously to induce sleep and also create a sense of calm peacefulness (provided, of course, that you are not allergic to the grains from which the toast is made).

To banish the blues permanently, increase the levels of raw food in your diet to between 50 and 75 percent each day. Try using the Juice Blitz one day each week for a few weeks as well, to help continue the detoxification process. Meanwhile, make your juices rich in dark green vegetables full of magnesium, potassium, iron, calcium and folic acid. A deficiency in any of these can contribute to depression, as can a deficiency in fatty acids, which is why it can be useful to add flaxseeds to your juices. Don't be discouraged if it takes a little time to deep cleanse your body and replenish the nutrients you may be lacking. It is well worth the effort.

Recipes that can help with depression include:
- Chlorophyll Plus
- Salsa Surprise
- Ginger Spice
- Hi Mag
- Red Genius
- Pineapple Special
- Linusit Perfect

DIGESTION

Digestive troubles come in many forms, from minor problems such as a bloated feeling after a meal, to abdominal pain and wind, nausea and more serious ailments like gastric ulcers, diverticulitis and colon troubles. In all these circumstances, it's important to avoid taking in any substances that can irritate the stomach, such as coffee, alcohol and chocolate. Occasionally, stomach troubles come from hypochlorhydria—a deficiency of hydrochloric acid—in which case pineapple and papaya juice are excellent since they are rich in protein digesting enzymes, bromelin and papain, respectively.

Among clinical reports of juicing, none is more impressive than the results that Dr. Garnett Cheney at Stanford University reported in his treatment of gastric ulcers using juices alone. Dr. Cheney prescribed for his patients fresh raw green cabbage juice, prepared and drunk immediately. It contains antipeptic ulcer factors which are really quite remarkable.

Leslie's mother, who was diagnosed with a peptic ulcer at the age of 37 and who was very resistant to taking any form of medication, read about Cheney's work and began to use cabbage juice. You need to swallow about five 8-ounce glasses a day, and she found that it worked superbly well: the ulcers cleared up and she never was troubled by them again.

Cabbage juice tends to benefit most digestive upsets. It's not exactly delicious, however, and it can be helpful to mix it with pineapple juice to soften the flavor. Ginger is also good for digestion and has been used for thousands of years to counteract nausea, travel sickness and morning sickness. Bananas have been shown to help protect the stomach from any excess of hydrochloric acid. Most people with any digestive upset that is not a serious medical condition requiring treatment find that simply getting into a Juice High way of living clears up the problem. These juices are especially good for that purpose:

- Pineappage
- Gingeroo
- Ginger Spice
- Red Flag
- Red Genius
- Tropical Prune

ECZEMA

An annoying condition that's often hard to get rid of, where the skin becomes red, swollen and itchy in the beginning then later thickens to produce crusted, scaly patches, eczema has many causes. Allergies are often a prime factor, which makes it important to use an elimination diet and to check for any food allergies. With eczema, as with any skin condition, it is important that your elimination works properly so that your skin is not forced to eliminate waste. Try the Juice Blitz and the High Life Diet.

Certain nutrients are also very important in eczema. Sweet peppers, tomatoes, cabbage and parsley are all excellent sources of bioflavonoids, which help improve inflammation and control allergy as well as enhance the capillaries so you get a better flow of nutrients and elimination of waste from the skin. Citrus fruits are also good, provided you incorporate the pithy, white covering inside the peel in your juices. Zinc is particularly important. It's usually found in good quantities in carrots, garlic, parsley and ginger. Carrots and parsley are also an excellent source of beta carotene, as are kale and spinach.

Recipes that can help with eczema include:
- Parsley Passion
- Spring Salad
- Gingeroo
- Green Wow
- Carrot & Apple
- Chlorophyll Plus

EYE HEALTH

The health of the eyes depends more than anything else on the quality of antioxidant protection that your body gets. Free-radical damage is a major factor in the development of both minor eye problems, such as short sightedness, to major problems, such as cataracts and glaucoma. For the eye to remain healthy, it needs to be able to maintain a normal balance and concentration of such minerals as calcium, potassium and sodium within the lens. When free-radical damage occurs, the cellular mechanisms by which nutrients are pumped to the eyes and excess sodium and wastes are removed from the eyes no longer work so well. Beta carotene, one of the most important of all of the bioflavonoids, is an antioxidant that helps protect the eye lens from ultraviolet damage.

Yellow, orange and dark green vegetables, which are rich in beta carotene as well as vitamins C and E, the B-complex, zinc, calcium and phosphorus, are very important for eye health. Ginger, garlic and parsley are rich in zinc, another mineral element that has been shown to be helpful. There is anecdotal evidence that drinking lots of carrot juice will improve eyesight, particularly night vision. Many aspiring pilots who found it difficult to pass the rigorous exams set to determine the quality of their vision have been able to improve their vision and pass the test by drinking lots and lots of carrot juice. Here are some of our favorite recipes for eyes:

- Spiked Celery
- Orange Tonic
- Double Whammy
- Pineapple Green
- Green Wild
- Hi Mag
- Carrot & Apple
- Beet Treat

FATIGUE

One of the underlying causes of fatigue, particularly in women, can be iron depletion. Spinach juice is a far better way of boosting iron levels than taking tablets, which tend to be highly constipating and are not really absorbed very well. The iron in natural foods and juices such as spinach, or any of the green leafy vegetables, and also in legumes, poultry, whole grains, liver and molasses, is highly bioavailable, i.e., your body has no trouble making use of it. Remember that replenishing the body of essential nutrients takes time; be prepared to work with natural foods and juices for several weeks before you start to see lasting results.

Make sure that 50 to 75 percent of the foods you each day are raw and make sure you get lots of chlorophyll rich foods. Cereal grasses are particularly good, as they are high in minerals, vitamins and enzymes and also have a wonderful ability to enliven the liver. Since most fatigue is the result of toxic build-up in the body, this helps to create more energy overall. Chlorophyll also helps protect from infectious diseases. When you are using wheat and barley-grass juice you can take it either as a supplement in powdered form that you add to your vegetables and fruit juices once they are made, or get a cereal grass juicer and grow your own cereal grasses (see Resources).

Magnesium is another important mineral when it comes to fatigue. Low intracellular magnesium makes the body very prone to infection, food allergies and chronic conditions. Good sources of magnesium are any of the dark green vegetables, whole grains, seaweeds, molasses, legumes, fish and nuts. These juice recipes are all beneficial:

- Dandelion Plus
- Parsley Passion
- Green Zinger
- Top of the Beet
- Ginger Berry
- Hi Mag

- Glorious Grapefruit
- Spinapple
- Secret of the Sea
- Sprout Special
- Atomic Lift-Off
- Hit the Grass
- Gingeroo
- Citrusucculent

HAIR LOSS

You may be genetically programmed to lose your hair, but that doesn't mean you have to let it go easily. There is a great deal you can do to prevent hair loss and, at the very least, slow it down dramatically. Eat more foods that are rich in sulphur, amino acids, L-methionine and L-cysteine. Eggs are a good, but when it comes to protection from hair loss, cabbage is king.

Be sure to cut out the foods that work against you. Sugars, for instance, will tend to increase the rate of hair loss, so try to eliminate sugar completely from your diet. Make sure to include in your diet plenty of foods that are rich in PABA, inositol and choline, such as mushrooms, spinach, legumes, lentils and brown rice. Consider adding a supplement of vacuum-packed flaxseeds to your diet. You can grind them in a coffee grinder and sprinkle them on salads or cereals in the morning. You can also add them to your juices.

Finally, the grain alfalfa has long been believed to stimulate hair growth, particularly in its sprouted form. Other juices that may be helpful include:

- Alfalfa—Father of All Juices
- Parsnip Perfect
- Fatty Acid Frolic

- Carrot High
- Spinapple
- Ginger's Best

HANGOVER

We all recognize that it's not a good idea to drink to excess, or to take drugs and go out dancing all night, but we're all liable to overenjoy ourselves every once in a while. The inevitable consequence of overindulgence is waking feeling dehydrated and nauseous, with a brain that feels like it's banging against the side of your head when you move. You need to replenish your bodily fluids, renutrify exhausted muscles and get your head together. Fruit juice is strongly indicated. Citrus juices, being full of natural sugar and vitamin C, are the most immediately effective remedy, but they may be a little harsh if your stomach is delicate. Watermelon, being exceptionally mild, is ideal.

There is an art to hangover management, and the key to it is regarding detoxification as the corollary of intoxication. All drugs provoke a strongly acidic reaction in the body, which causes the symptoms of a hangover, and the first step to recovery is to correct the body's chemical imbalance. Plain old Carrot and Apple juice is effective for rebalancing and it's easy to take when you're feeling weak. By incorporating beet juice, you will greatly assist the repair of any possible damage done to your liver and kidneys.

Recipes that can help with hangovers include:
- Merry Belon
- Beet Treat
- Apple & Pear
- Carrot & Apple

INSOMNIA

Insomnia can have many causes. Drugs that you might be taking, such as beta-blockers or thyroid medication, or even caffeine and alcohol can all disrupt sleep. So, ironically, can sleeping pills if your body becomes addicted to them.

Getting regular exercise—that is, long walks, not going to aerobics classes and throwing your back out of place—can help enormously to reduce the nervous tension that prevents sleep. Sometimes sleep is disrupted by hypoglycemia, so make sure you don't have a blood sugar problem (see *Low Blood Sugar*, page 135). Eliminate coffee, tea, alcohol and junk foods—including diet colas—from your life once and for all. Eat your biggest meal at lunchtime, as everyone sleeps better (and longer) when their stomach is not full. Consider using one of the well-proven natural tranquilizers such as Valerian, Passiflora (Passion flower), Wild Lettuce. You can make a nightcap cocktail to help increase the levels of serotonin in the brain, a sleep-inducing neurotransmitter in the brain, and blend into it one capful or a pinch of Valerian, Passiflora or Wild Lettuce (see Resources for suppliers).

Certain nutrients are particularly important too, such as magnesium, vitamin B6 and niacin, simply because they have to be present in order for the amino acid tryptophan to be able to turn itself into serotonin. Carrots are a rich source of all three. Calcium is also important in inducing muscle relaxation, and so is folic acid, which, in sufficient quantities, prevents leg twitching (called Restless Leg Syndrome) and nervous tension from building in the body. The green drinks, from dandelion to parsley and spinach, are excellent sources of folic acid and calcium. Seaweed is also a very good source of magnesium. Many people need an extra boost of fruit sugar (not, however, if you have a low blood sugar problem) before going to bed to trigger sleep. Pineapple and grape is a wonderful combination for this. Others include:

- Spicy Carrot
- Hi Mag
- Green Goddess
- Pineapple Special
- Sprout Special
- Pineamint
- Lazy Lettuce
- Smooth as Silk

LOW BLOOD SUGAR (HYPOGLYCEMIA)

Low blood sugar—where the body tends to secrete insulin, which in turn makes the blood sugar level drop, depriving the brain of its main "food," glucose—is a condition that underlies much of the chocolate-munching and coffee-drinking in which people tend to indulge in order to keep themselves going.

When there are disturbances in insulin and blood sugar production, the balance of hormones in the body is upset and can produce and enormous number of periodic symptoms including palpitations of the heart, sweating, depression, anxiety, headaches, poor concentration and bad temper. These symptoms are alleviated by munching on some sort of carbohydrate, such as a slice of whole-grain bread. The trick in clearing up the condition, however, is to clear out of your life everything that would trigger the pancreas to oversecrete insulin. In particular this means no sugar, chocolate or bottled fruit juices. Choose foods that are rich in complex carbohydrates and fiber, such as raw vegetables, whole oats, beans, whole-grain pasta, lentils, chickpeas, etc. Sprouted seeds are particularly good.

The vegetable juices are better than the fruit juices until blood sugar is stabilized. Don't drink fruit juices unless they are well diluted with mineral water, and then only a couple of times a week. Try adding a little turmeric or cinnamon to your juices. Both these spices have long been used to help stabilize blood sugar. Use foods which are rich in chromium, which helps regulate glucose metabolism in the body, such as spinach, apples, green peppers, whole grains, clams and liver, as well as foods which are rich in manganese, such as carrots, celery, beet, beet greens, turnip greens, pineapple, liver, eggs, green vegetables and buckwheat.

An antidote for a sweet tooth is lots of green drinks, but you will have to get yourself used to drinking them since they are about the last thing that the hypoglycemic wants. Once you do get used to them, you will find that your blood sugar stabilizes and you have energy to spare, day in and day out. All of the green juices are excellent, such as:

- Green Friend
- Parsley Passion
- Green Zinger
- Dandelion Plus
- Secret of the Sea
- Lemon Zinger
- Spicy Apple
- Tossled Carrot

MIGRAINE

When Leslie was 25 years old, she met a doctor who taught her about supporting the body to heal itself using juices and raw foods. Dr. Philip Kilsby had 99 percent success in the treatment of migraine, using juices, lots of raw fruits and vegetables, and a few dietary supplements. The only case of migraine he could not cure was a woman who turned out not to have migraine but a brain tumor.

Kilsby taught that all migraines—regardless of whether the cause is a possible food allergy, a chemical allergy, stress-related, and so forth—are centered in a liver that is overworked, trying to keep the body internally clear. One of the major things in the treatment of migraine that Kilsby did was to take all the stress off the liver by removing from the diet foods containing tyramine, as well as other foods that people are commonly allergic to, such as red wine, other alcohol, salad dressings, red plums, soft cheeses, figs, aged game, chicken liver, canned meat, salami, pickled herring, eggplant, soy sauce, yeast concentrates, as well as other foods that are commonly known to trigger food allergy such as chocolate, wheat, milk, the food coloring tartrazine, sugar, coffee and peanuts.

He then put his patients on a detox program very much like the Juice Blitz, followed by the High Life Diet. Dr. Kilsby found that once patients started on the program they usually experienced another migraine while the body was detoxifying, then maybe yet a further one or two, each one milder than the last one, until—provided they looked after their diet—the migraines disappeared altogether. Kilsby insisted his patients drink a juice rich in green vegetables twice daily.

Migraines are known to be triggered by the contraction followed by a quick dilation of the blood vessels in the brain, all things that can be triggered by certain foods. Biofeedback can be helpful for some people where they train themselves to visualize their hands as warm, thereby drawing blood away from the head and taking pressure off the area that is involved in the migraine. The herb feverfew can also be useful to many people.

If you suffer from migraines, you want to leave out of your diet all chemicals, including artificial sweeteners such as aspartame. You might also consider including in your juices some of the fruits and vegetables which are known to reduce platelet stickiness since foods that inhibit blood clotting are known to reduce migraine. These include garlic, cantaloupe and ginger.

Recipes that can help with migranes include:

- Green Goddess
- Spring Salad
- Gingeroo
- Dandelion Plus
- Green Friend
- Sprout Special

PROSTATE TROUBLE

Enlargement of the prostate is so common that 60 percent of men between the ages of 40 to 59 have the condition, which is properly known as Benign Prostatic Hyperplasia (BPH). When this occurs, there is an obstruction of the bladder outlet, increased frequency of urination and difficulty in urinating. The standard medical treatment for BPH is surgery. However, there is a great deal that can be done to improve the condition through nutrition. BPH is a hormone-dependent disorder of the metabolism. Testosterone, especially free-testosterone levels, decreases after age 55. Meanwhile other hormones such as oestradiol, luteinizing hormone and follicle-stimulating hormone, as well as prolactin, all increase. This in effect leads to an increased concentration of a very potent male hormone called dihydrotestosterone within the prostate itself, which is responsible for the overproduction of prostate cells. This ultimately results in the enlarged prostate.

Protecting yourself against high levels of female hormone mimics, or xeno-hormones, from the environment (petrochemical derivatives which are taken up by receptor sites in the body and mimic the effect of the estrogens) is an important part of diminishing prostate enlargement. As is decreasing levels of prolactin. Prolactin levels are increased by both stress and beer, therefore these are two things that need to be eliminated, while the mineral zinc and vitamin B6 have been shown to reduce prolactin levels yet produce no side effects in reasonable doses. Zinc has been shown to reduce the size of the prostate and to reduce symptoms in men who suffer from BPH. Similarly, essential fatty acids such as those found in organic flaxseed or flaxseed oil have been shown to bring about a significant improvement in many patients with the condition.

It is important that the patient is protected as much as possible from pesticides, herbicides and other petrochemically derived compounds in the environment such as biphenyls, hexachlorobenzene and dioxin, which can increase the formation of dihidrotestosterone in the prostate. Go for juices that are high in zinc and B6 and drinks containing organically grown, vacuum-packed flaxseeds. These are among the best:

- Ginger Spice
- Pineapple Green
- Ginger's Best
- Silky Strawberries
- Green Friend
- Green Zinger
- Dandelion Plus
- Linusit Perfect

PREMENSTRUAL SYNDROME

PMS comes in many forms and causes many symptoms, from irritability, depression, tension and decreased energy, to backache, breast pain, changes in libido, abdominal bloating, edema and headache. It has been divided into four basic groups, depending upon the symptoms, each of which has specific biochemical needs, deficiencies and patterns in common. However, there are certain things that all PMS sufferers need to watch. It is essential to clear sugar out of your diet as well as cut down any other form of refined carbohydrates, including white flour and honey. Avoid coffee, tea and chocolate, for two reasons—first because they contain methylxanthines, which have been linked with a number of the symptoms associated with PMS. Secondly, because anything containing caffeine can have a very negative effect on such things as breast tenderness, anxiety and depression.

It is also a good idea to eliminate all milk products and wheat from your diet for seven days prior to menstruation. At the same time there are certain nutrients that are important to emphasize: magnesium, B6 and the B-complex, particularly B6, as well as beta carotene. Bromelin, too, can be helpful since this enzyme is believed to help relax the smooth muscle tissue of the body. Go for the green juices, which are rich in all these things. If you have water retention, turn toward watermelon, grape, cucumber and dandelion, each of which has a splendid ability to eliminate excess water from the system. You are likely to find that all of the juices that are good for PMS are also useful for someone who is wrestling with menopausal symptoms such as hot flashes. For both PMS and menopausal symptoms, it can be enormously helpful to follow a Raw Energy way of eating where 50 to 75 percent of your foods are taken raw during the 7 to 10 days before a period or whenever the symptoms seem to be at their worst. Here are some of the most useful recipes for PMS:

- Hi Mag
- Ginger Berry
- Pineapple Special
- Pineapple Green
- Spring Salad
- Waterfall
- Cool as a Cuke
- Black Watermelon
- Green Zinger
- Secret of the Sea
- Sprout Special

STRESS

Stress is a complicated condition to treat since it can have so many causes and take so many forms. However, whenever the body is under prolonged stress certain things happen— a major one being that the tissues of the body tend to become more acidic. There is nothing better to do when your system is too acidic than to drink fresh vegetable and fruit juices to alkalinize it. As you do this you will find your whole experience of life changes. Detoxification, too, helps eliminate the sense of constant tension, anxiety and frustration that so often goes with stress, as well as with any of the physical complaints that come in its wake, from gastrointestinal difficulties, high blood pressure and dizziness to loss of appetite or excessive appetite and headaches.

While it is important to practice some sort of deep relaxation or meditation if you are suffering from prolonged stress, the effect of dietary change alone, incorporating a Juice High regime into your lifestyle and making between 50 and 75 percent of your foods raw, can literally transform your life within two weeks. There are certain nutrients that are particularly useful in strengthening your body's ability to handle stress, such as pantothenic acid, which occurs in good quantity in green leafy vegetables such as kale, dandelion and broccoli; potassium, which is found in good quantity in bananas, parsley and spinach; zinc, good sources of which are carrots and ginger; and magnesium, which also occurs in good quantity in the green foods. All these juices are useful:

- Silky Strawberries
- Easy Does It
- Gingeroo
- Hi Mag
- Ginger Spice
- Green Friend
- Hit the Grass
- Sprout Special

SKIN TROUBLES

Whether you are counteracting acne, aging or eczema, when it comes to improving the health of skin, you have to look to your diet. Eliminate all hydrogenated fats such as margarines and use extra-virgin olive oil instead. Also, avoid fried foods, coffee, chocolate and tea, and get yourself into a good detox program like the Juice Blitz followed by the High Life Diet.

Most skin problems are influenced by an inability in the body to eliminate waste fully through other channels such as the urine and feces. Therefore wastes get clogged within the system and the body attempts to eliminate them through the skin. Then you end up with pimples, acne, or simply lackluster, aging skin. Blitzing often clears this up easily, although it must be said that in the first day or so the skin conditions can become worse as the body is eliminating them before they get better.

Carrot juice, high in beta carotene, is absolutely brilliant for skin. So are all the green drinks, which are rich in folic acid. Finally, raw flaxseed added to your drinks will give great support to skin, no matter what the specific problem you are trying to eliminate.

Recipes that can help with skin problems include:
- Raw NRG
- Ginger Spice
- Red Cool
- Green Zinger
- Hi Mag
- Tropical Prune
- Dandelion Plus
- Tossled Carrot
- Sprout Special
- Linusit Perfect

URINARY INFECTIONS

Cranberry juice is excellent for any sort of kidney and urinary infections. Cranberry is also thought to be good for an underactive thyroid, partly because many of the bogs in which cranberries are grown, particularly in the United States, are near the ocean and rich in iodine, which the fruit absorb. Cranberry juice on its own is much too strong for most people to handle. However, it mixes beautifully with any number of gentler juices like melon or apple. It will also add extra zest to basic vegetable juices like carrot. Cranberry is known for its cleansing properties, helping to rid not only the digestive system but also other organs of the body of waste and bacteria. It is also said to be very good for skin problems such as acne. A useful recipe for urinary infection is:

- Cranberry Cocktail

WATER RETENTION

Water retention is a sign that your body is sluggish at eliminating waste, that the metabolism is not working properly and the body needs to be deep cleansed and rebalanced. It can be caused by many things, from hormones in birth control pills and hormone replacement therapy to hormone changes during the premenstruum and pregnancy. It can also be caused by food allergies and liver problems.

Encouraging the body to eliminate excess water from its tissues is a two-fold process. First, use natural diuretics such as nettle, dill, watermelon, grapes and cucumber that gently encourage the loss of excess water. Second, detoxify the system as a whole using the Juice Blitz. If swelling in the ankles is severe and prolonged, it can indicate serious problems such as heart failure, so you need to check with your doctor. It is good to check for any possibility of food allergy if you have prolonged water retention and to decrease the amount of salt in your diet. The sodium/ potassium balance in your body determines to a great extent whether the body eliminates excess fluids properly. Eliminate sugar from your diet.

One of the major things that you can do to help your body eliminate water retention is increase the number of potassium-rich foods that you eat and make your juices from. These include: bananas, prunes, raisins, figs, seaweeds, fish, green vegetables, whole grains, kale, broccoli, spinach, Swiss chard, and all the other green foods, plus carrot and celery. You may be deficient in vitamin B6, which can interfere with the kidneys' ability to eliminate waste. Foods rich in B6 include molasses, brown rice, liver, eggs, cabbage and fish. Garlic, too, is one of the traditional foods for eliminating edema from the tissues.

Recipes that can help with water retention include:

- Cool as a Cuke
- Black Watermelon
- Potassium Power
- Green Friend
- Green Zinger
- Dandelion Plus
- Secret of the Sea

9

GREEN LIGHTNING

Once you get the basics of juicing under your belt—and once you get used to the wild, raw taste of fresh vegetables—you are ready for the next step: green lightning. And what a step it is. Green juices, like the foods they are pressed from, are little short of magical. They bring you increased energy, protection from radiation in the environment and from degenerative diseases, as well as enhanced immune performance. Green foods will even help regenerate and rejuvenate the body. Go green and you can wave those annoying winter colds and flus goodbye. The old adage "eat your greens if you want to stay young and healthy" is now scientific fact. And the fun of it all is that, so far, advanced nutritional scientists know that green works wonders, but nobody is yet sure why. The chlorophyll? The enzymes? Mystery ingredients? Yes, probably, but maybe other reasons too. The very latest nutritional supplements have gone green—spirulina, chlorella, green barley, blue-green algae. Why? Because the nutrients they contain—from vitamins and minerals to trace elements, enzymes and as yet unidentified health-promoting factors are not only richest in green foods, they are found there in perfect balance and synergy as well as in a highly bioavailable form. Your system just laps them up.

Bountiful Brassicas

Dark green vegetables such as broccoli, Brussels sprouts, collards, kale, kohlrabi and mustard greens have hit the headlines in the last few years thanks to an overwhelming abundance of medical and scientific evidence that they help prevent cancer. Prestigious medical journals such as the *Journal of the National Cancer Institute* and *Federation Proceedings* report, for instance, that the sulphur and histidine in these brassicas—members of the cabbage family— inhibit the growth of cancer tumors, detoxify the system of poisonous environmental channels, prevent colon cancer and increase the body's own supply of natural cancer-fighting compounds. They can also help lower low-density lipoproteins—the *bad* cholesterol—which accompanies hardening of the arteries. They improve elimination and fight yeast infections, too. Adding a couple of florets of broccoli or a few leaves of kale to a glass of carrot juice turns something good into something even better. But start slow and gradually build up on the green. In the beginning—especially if you have a sweet tooth or if you are addicted to sugar—the taste can seem pretty strong. Then build up gradually until you find that your old craving for sugars has actually been transformed into a new craving for green.

Grass That's Greener

Another group of green lightning foods, the cereal grasses, are some of the least known but most powerful green foods. You need special equipment to extract the juice from them, but these grasses are sold in health food stores as a dried powder and can be stirred into raw juice by the teaspoon full. The grasses have been around for thousands of years, however only in the last 10 or 15 years has the consumption of young grass—wheat or rye or oat or barley—begun to rise. In ancient times, of course, young cereal plants were treated with the respect they deserve. Tiny green tips of baby wheat plants were eaten as a delicacy in the Holy Land 2000 years ago. In the 1920s and 30s, before vitamin and mineral pills were in existence, bottled, dehydrated cereal grass became a popular food supplement in the West.

Young grasses are very different from the mature grains they eventually turn into, from which we make our breads and cereals. Dark green in color, in some ways they are similar to dark green brassica vegetables in their protective abilities. But they are very special, too. When rice, wheat, corn, oats, barley, rye or millet are planted in good healthy soil with plenty of rainfall and are harvested at exactly the right moment, not only do they taste sweet, but are unbelievably rich in vitamins and minerals, enzymes and growth hormones you would be hard-pressed to find elsewhere. They are living foods, and the juice pressed from them carries these life energies into your body. The young germinated plant is a little miracle of nature. In the young leaves, photosynthesis produces simple sugars which they transform into proteins, fatty acids, nucleic acids such as DNA and RNA, as well as complex carbohydrates, thanks to the work of enzymes and substrates produced from minerals provided by the soil. The peak of nutritional bounty in all cereal grasses—the moment when chlorophyll, protein and most of the vitamins and minerals reach their zenith—occurs just before *jointing*. This is the moment at which the young internodal tissue in the grass leaf starts to elongate and form a stem. This is when cereal grasses are best harvested. It is usually somewhere between 8 and 15 days after planting. Afterward, the chlorophyll, protein and vitamin content drops dramatically while the fiber content increases rapidly. To give you some idea of just how remarkable the nutritional content of young cereal grasses can be it is useful to compare, say, fresh wheatgrass to freshly milled whole-wheat flour:

GREEN BLOOD

Serious research into the effects of feeding animals and humans on young green cereal plants has gone on for three quarters of a century. In 1928, chemist Charles Schnabel was searching for some material that could be added to poultry feeds to improve egg production and lower chicken mortality. He wanted what he described as a "blood building-material." Before long, scientists had discovered that chlorophyll—the green substance in plants—has a remarkable similarity in its chemical structure to hemoglobin—the oxygen-carrying factor in animal blood. Schnabel figured that magic "green leaves should be the best source of blood." So he began to feed all sorts of green things to chickens—from alfalfa to combinations of twenty green vegetables. But he found them all lacking. Then he tried giving hens a greens mixture that "just happened to contain a large amount of immature wheat and oats." Animals who got only 10 percent of this cereal grass responded amazingly. Winter egg production shot up from an average of 38 percent to 94 percent of summer levels, and the eggs that were produced had stronger shells, hatching healthier chicks.

Intrigued by his success with chickens, Schnable began to investigate every aspect of cereal grasses—from the soils that produce the most nutritionally rich grasses to the effect that giving dehydrated grasses has on the health of humans. He also fed his own family of seven on the grasses and was known to boast that none of them ever had a serious illness or a decayed tooth. He even developed a vision of how to feed the hungry of the world on the exceedingly high-quality protein from cereal grasses.

THE GRASS JUICE FACTOR

In the decades that followed, other scientists working with animal nutrition, such as Dr. George Kohler at University of Wisconsin and Dr. Mott Cannon at University of Cali-

NUTRIENTS PER 100 GRAMS DRY WEIGHT		
	Wheatgrass	**Whole-Wheat Flour**
Chlorophyll (mg)	543	0
Vitamin A (IU)	23,136	0
Total Dietary Fiber (g)	37	10
Protein (g)	32	13
Carbohydrates (g)	37	71
Calcium (mg)	277	41
Vitamin C	51	0
Iron	34	4
Folic Acid (mcg)	100	38
Niacin (mg)	6.1	4.3
Riboflavin (mg)	2.03	0.12

fornia at Berkeley, confirmed that a mixture of young cereal grasses fed to livestock improved milk production in cows and produced stronger more resilient, longer-living animals all around—from guinea pigs and rats to rabbits, cats and ferrets. Others discovered that green cereal grass feeds, which are believed to contain natural plant steroid hormones, both enhanced fertility and improved lactation in all manner of animals including humans. Since then, scientists have done their best to isolate and identify the ingredient or ingredients in young cereal grasses responsible for all of this. But to this day, the amazing "grass juice factor" has not been identified.

That has not, however, stopped people from making practical use of it. Take Ann Wigmore, a raw food enthusiast. She had seen her grandmother give young grasses to help heal wounded soldiers in the First World War. When she herself became ill, she began to experiment with growing grasses—especially wheatgrasses—to help heal herself. The results were astounding. Her long-standing and medically untreatable colitis cleared; her hair, which had gone gray, returned to its natural dark color. Her energy levels soared. Full of enthusiasm, after a few months she started to give juice pressed from young cereal grasses to her animals, her neighbors and others who had heard of what it could do. In 1968 she founded Hippocrates Health Institute in Boston—a treatment and educational center for people with chronic degenerative conditions where she evangelized the use of wheatgrass and wheatgrass juice therapies as well as green and raw foods. Wigmore claimed that immature grasses are effective in treating an enormous variety of ailments, from obesity and chronic fatigue to ulcers, liver and pancreatic problems, high blood pressure and certain cancers, as well as asthma, anemia, hemorrhoids, skin troubles, constipation and eczema. Now, if you were to do a computer search of the most up-to-date medical and scientific literature, you would find many animal studies and much clinical research to support her assertions.

EASTERN PROMISE

Around the same time, a Japanese research chemist Yoshihide Hagiwara also suffered from ill health. He also began to explore the nutritional powers of cereal grasses after conventional treatments proved of no avail. He eventually found that he was able to heal himself by radically changing his diet and using Chinese herbs. Then, convinced that there must be thousands of other people who suffered as he had, Hagiwara began to investigate numerous health-promoting natural foods. After several years of experimenting, he came to the conclusion that "the leaves of cereal grasses provide the nearest thing to the perfect food that this planet offers." But where Wigmore had concentrated on the uses of wheatgrass, Hagiwara focused his efforts on green barley. Given juice extracts of barley grass, animals and humans appear to experience the same kind of health enhancement reported by Wigmore. Hagiwara has confirmed the ability of barley grass juice to lower serum cholesterol, while the work of other Japanese scientists has isolated two interesting proteins that enhance health and stimulate healing. P4-D1 and D1-G1 might yet prove to be the keys to the "grass juice factor."

P4-D1 was found to have an ability to protect cells from ultraviolet radiation and from specific cancer-causing substances. Researchers who have worked with it believe this is probably the result of the protein's ability to stimulate the repair of DNA. If this turns out to be the case, it may in part explain the reported ability that young cereal grasses have to rejuvenate an organism. Since damage to DNA is a major factor in aging, if this turns out to be the case, it could go some way to explaining the reported ability that young cereal grasses have to rejuvenate an organism. But it is likely that there are other factors at work, too. At the Linus Pauling Institute at Oregon State University, researchers investigating skin cancer found that by feeding vitamin C to mice, they could reduce the incidence of the disease five fold. However, when the mice were fed on a diet made up only of fruits, wheatgrass, carrots and sunflower seeds they witnessed a 35-fold decrease in skin cancer. Another researcher, Dr. Chiu Nan Lai, verified that wheatgrass might have anticancer properties. She demonstrated that when an extract of wheatgrass is applied to cancer causing chemicals this would decrease the ability of mutagens to trigger cancer by as much as 99 percent.

QUANTUM SUNLIGHT

One well-known health-promoting ingredient in young cereal grasses and green foods is chlorophyll—the stuff that makes plants green. The chlorophyll molecule is unique in the universe. It is the only thing that has the ability to convert the energy of the sun into chemical energy through the mysterious process of photosynthesis. It is thanks to the chlorophyll molecule that plants make carbohydrates out of carbon dioxide and water. All of life on earth draws its power to be from the sun's energy thanks to photosynthesis in plants. The molecular design of chlorophyll is built around a central structure known as a porphyrin ring. It is the same structure which molecules involved in the transportation of oxygen and cellular respiration in our own body have at their center. The most important of these is hemoglobin—the substance that carries oxygen from the lungs to other tissues in the body via the red blood cells. The main difference between hemoglobin and chlorophyll is that where the molecular structure of chlorophyll has magnesium at its center, that of the heme molecule in hemoglobin has iron.

This similarity was first documented in the 19th century, and for many years some scientists, observing that animals who ate lots of green plants had plenty of hemoglobin in their red blood cells, believed that the reason why chlorophyll-filled plants were so good at "building blood" was that the two molecules were virtually interchangeable. Now, after more than 75 years of investigating why chlorophyll-rich plants are so good for the health of man, most scientists have come to believe that it is probably the synergistic effect of the chlorophyll and the vital nutrients—both known and unknown—found together with it in the plants from which it comes including iron, copper, calcium, magnesium, pyridoxine folic acid, vitamin C, B12, K and A. It would appear to be one of those situations when the *whole* of which chlorophyll is an important ingredient is far greater than any of its parts. H. E. Kirchner, MD, who spent many years investigating the power of cereal grasses and green foods, has written, "Chlorophyll, the healer, is at once powerful and bland—devastating to germs, yet gentle to wounded body tissues. Exactly how it works is still Nature's secret; to the layman, at least, the phenomenon seems like green magic." No wonder for thousands of years the leaves and green stems of plants have been used for supporting detoxification of the body, wound-healing, deodorization and any number of other beneficial effects.

Environmental Protector
In many experiments chlorophyll has been shown to pro-

tect animals from gene mutations associated with cancer through exposure to dangerous chemicals such as benzopyrene and methylcholanthrene. It is also known to inhibit the carcinogenic effects of exposure to simpler environmental poisons such as coal dust, tobacco and to foods such as red wine and fried beef. In fact, chlorophyll used on its own for these purposes has been proved to be more effective than antioxidant vitamins, A, C and E. Simple chlorophyll also helps protect from radiation. And when two or more of the dark green vegetables and cereal grasses are used together, an animal's resistance to radiation reaches a peak. Chlorophyll also inhibits the growth of bacteria by creating an environment in which they simply do not reproduce. It also decreases swelling and reduces inflammation and speeds wound healing while reducing itching, irritation and pain. When it comes to peptic ulcers, the chlorophyll-rich green juices come into their own as they do in the treatment of constipation, spastic colitis, halitosis and a number of other conditions.

Ask Any Weed

Some of the very best of the green foods to add to your raw energy juices are the weeds—plants that grow wild in your garden or in fields and hedgerows of the country. Weeds such as dandelion and nettles, ragweed and lambsquarter, are especially good sources of the minerals that our bodies have become depleted of as a result of chemical farming which has removed them from the subsoil. This is especially important when it comes to trace elements. Plants such as nettles only grow on mineral-rich soils. Weeds are deep feeders. They are capable of absorbing through their root systems all sorts of goodness that crops cultivated on depleted soils have no access to, and they store up valuable nutrients in a wonderful balance—ideal for the body to make use of. A handful of young nettles (they don't sting yet) is a great boon to a glass of carrot and apple juice. In addition to all of these things which weeds have in common, each plant is unique in the goodness it offers when added to a glass of juice. Dandelion, like nettle, is a natural diuretic—which is why in French its common name is *pis en lit*—and a blood cleanser and is stunningly rich in the carotenoids. Lambsquarter, a wayside spring and summer plant, is not only rich in minerals thanks to being a particularly "deep diver," it also tastes delicious and can be used in salads as well as juices without ever imparting too heavy a green flavor. Comfrey added to fresh juice (in small quantities) is rich in allantoin, which herbalists have long used to soothe intestinal irritations from stomach ulcers to diarrhea as well as to calm skin eruptions and heal wounds.

Seaweeds are another great additive to juicing. You can use them in the form of powdered kelp, dried nori, arame, hiziki, laver bread, dulse, kombu and wakami. Seaweeds are full of trace elements which are needed by the body only in minute quantities, and yet when they are not there can create big holes in energy and body functioning—things like boron, chromium, cobalt, calcium, iodine, magnesium, manganese, molybdenum, phosphorus, potassium, silicon, solver and sulphur, to mention only a few. Unlike the chalk, which is added to bread to "enrich" it with calcium, and most of the mineral supplements you by in pill form in stores, the minerals in green plants such as these are organic, which means that your body can easily make use of them to build health.

The Ultragreens

Watercress and parsley are two common green foods that are superb additions to your juices. They are ultragreen and very powerful, so you need very little to get a lot of benefit from them. Watercress contains lots more organic minerals than spinach and is richer in vitamins, too. It has a high sulphur content, which experts in natural medicine claim helps to improve the functioning of the endocrine system. Thanks to its iron, manganese and copper content, it is also known to be good for strengthening the blood and eliminating anemia. It is also rich in vitamins C and E. Parsley is another natural diuretic—great for cleansing the body of wastes and reducing edema. It is famous for its ability to improve the health of the kidneys and for its antioxidant compounds including masses of beta carotene. Like watercress juice, parsley juice is superpotent both in taste and in actions—you need only a stalk or two of either plant to rev up any juice you are making, turning it into a green powerhouse.

Good, Better, Best

It is easy when looking at the power of green juices—which concentrate the health-promoting abilities of plants as nothing else can—to get lost in fascination with research into what they offer in the way of help for sick people. Far more important is what green lightning can offer to those of us who are already well but would like to feel better, be leaner and have even more energy. For of all the combinations of fruit and vegetable juices, the greens are the great powerhouse. You can go green in three ways. First, you can add a handful—make it small at first until you get into green juicing—of kale, broccoli or dark green cabbage to a simple base such as half carrot and half apple. Second—and better still—you can grow organic cereal grasses like wheatgrass or barley in trays and harvest as you need them, but you will need special equipment to juice them, as described in the resources section at the back of the book, to add to your vegetable juices. Finally, you can buy freeze-dried wheatgrass or green barley, or one of the other green magic foods such as spirulina or chlorella—more about them in a moment—to whatever juice you feel like.

Growing cereal grasses can be fun if you love nurturing things and looking after them. For most of us with busy lives, however, the green powders are easiest and best, provided of course that they are organic, fresh and properly prepared. (See Resources for how to sprout grasses, what to buy in powder form and where to get it.)

MAGIC SPIRALS

Not only can cereal grasses be found in easy-to-use powdered form to stir into your juices, so can other highly nutritious natural green additives such as seaweeds and chlorella. Use them freely. They will do you nothing but good. Queen of them all is spirulina. A near-microscopic form of blue-green freshwater algae, spirulina is one of the finest green additives to your juices that you will ever find. It is made up of translucent, bubble-thin cells stacked end to end to form an incredibly beautiful deep green helix. Spirulina is but one specific form of blue-green algae of which there are more than 25,000 varieties on the planet. Back 3.5 billion years ago, these plants began to fix nitrogen from the atmosphere and to convert it into carbon dioxide and sugars and in the process to release free oxygen. This created the oxygen-rich atmosphere in which the rest of life was able to develop.

Spirulina is remarkable in so many ways that it is hard to list them all. It is probably the single most important nutritional supplement you can use to support health at the very highest level. Rich in easy-to-assimilate protein, it has a superior amino acid profile. It is unusual in that its protein is alkaline-forming in the body rather than acid-forming. This can be very important for detoxifying the system and also for helping you deal with high levels of stress. For the byproducts of prolonged stress tend to be acid in character and spirulina, like fresh vegetables juices themselves being alkaline, helps to neutralize them. Spirulina is also rich in vitamins E, B12, C, B1, B5 and B6 as well as beta carotene and the minerals zinc, copper, manganese and selenium. It also contains good levels of the antiaging antioxidant sulphur amino acid methionine and *phycocyanin*—a blue pigment structurally similar to beta carotene which experiments have shown enhance immune functions. Finally, it is rich in important essential fatty acids, although it's very low in fat. Add from a teaspoon to a tablespoon to a grass of fresh juice or mix a glass of fresh juice together with spirulina and a banana in a blender for a great breakfast drink.

EMERALD TREASURE

Chlorella, sometimes called the emerald food, is another green algae with pretty amazing properties that is great as a juice additive. It gets its name from its high content of chlorophyll—the highest of any known plant. In addition, it is rich in vitamins, minerals, fiber, nucleic acids, amino acids, enzymes, something called CGF—chlorella growth factor—and other important compounds. Chlorella is the biggest-selling health food supplement in Japan. It has a very strong cell wall, which prevented us from making good use of its richness until 1977, when a process was developed to make chlorella into a powder without destroying its goodness. Among the green foods, chlorella is known as the great normalizer thanks to its apparent ability to alter bodily processes that are underactive or overactive so that they return to normal. About 60 percent of chlorella is protein. The vitamins it contains in good quantity include vitamin C, beta carotene and other carotenoids, thiamine, riboflavin, pyridoxine, niacin, pantothenic acid, folic acid, vitamin B12, biotin, choline, vitamin K, inositol and PABA. In addition, it is rich in minerals and trace elements, including phosphorus, potassium, magnesium, sulphur, iron, calcium, manganese, copper, zinc and cobalt.

In the seventies, scientists in Japan carrying out animal studies with chlorella discovered that it has an ability to stimulate the production of white blood cells and enhance immunity as well as having antiviral activity. It is also a powerful food for detoxifying the body. It can bind heavy metals such as cadmium, pesticide and herbicide poisons including PCB, and help remove them from the body. Meanwhile it helps protect the liver from toxic injury so well that some practitioners who use it claim it can even help prevent hangovers by promoting the removal of alcohol from the body.

Easy Does It

The secret with using any of the green lightning foods—from crunchy broccoli to wheatgrass or spirulina—is to begin small and keep adding as you get used to the green. Generally speaking, the worse your diet has been before you begin, the less you will like the taste of the green foods in the beginning. This is particularly true if you have always been a big sugar eater. Green lightning and sugar are at the opposite ends of the food continuum. This may be one of the reasons why going green with your juices is about the best thing you can do to counter low blood sugar, low energy problems or Candida albicans. Once you get used to green, you will love not only the way it makes you feel and look but even the way it tastes—so fresh and clean and alive.

Quantum Green Drink

Many of the green foods are strong in their plant structures and therefore can be difficult to break down in a juicer. That is why when using watercress or parsley or one of the weeds, instead of popping them into the juicer along with the carrots or celery or apples, we prefer to put the green food into a blender and pulverize it quickly then add our freshly made glass of juice and whisk again for no more than a few seconds before drinking. This way you produce a therapeutic green drink that is equal to none. Dr. H. E. Kirchner, one of the world experts on the use of green foods and grasses for health, has always insisted that such green drinks are the basis of preventative nutrition. We have learned much from him. Here is our version of his famous "Green Drink." We call it Quantum Green.

Make a glass of carrot and apple juice or fresh pineapple juice. Pour it into a blender and add a handful of sunflower seeds that have been soaked in spring water overnight as well as half the quantity of almonds and five dates without their seeds. Now put in a handful or two of green leaves or sprouted green foods such as alfalfa or mung beans. Choose from comfrey, lambsquarter, dandelion, parsley, mint, watercress, kale, or beet top—using the leaves only, never the stems. Now liquefy the greens by blending for a few moments. Made with sunflower seeds and almonds, this is a rich protein food ideal for a meal replacement any time. If you want a lower-protein drink, leave out the seeds and nuts or cut their quantities in half.

Here are some more of our favorite green recipes. Experiment with them and see what you come up with for yourself. Then let us know. We are always eager to find new ways of playing with green lightning.

Pineapple Green

This is a great way to wake up.

To a glass of freshly pressed pineapple juice, add one or more of the following:
1 tsp to 1 tbsp of powdered wheatgrass, green barley, spirulina or chlorella

Green Goddess

This juice makes you smile like the Mona Lisa.

1 carrot
1 apple
1/2 beet
2 florets broccoli
1 tsp kelp powder
1 tsp of chopped fresh parsley
a squeeze of fresh lemon juice

Juice as usual and serve.

Leslie's Cocktail

Rich and filling, this will carry you through the morning hunger-free.

2 apples
1 ripe banana
1 tsp each spirulina, chlorella and green barley powder

Green Wow

2 green apples
1 globe of fennel
4 stalks of celery
6 bok choy leaves
juice of half a cucumber

Sprouting o' the Green

This offers great protection from environmental-pollution damage and is quite delicious at the same time.

2 cups alfalfa sprouts
2 cups mung bean sprouts
1 carrot
a few sprigs parsley
2 apples

10

JUICE FREEDOM

We have examined the biochemical effect living juices have on the body, we have looked at the practicality of juicing and all the rites and rituals of deep cleansing and energizing the body. But what ultimately is it all about? What can you expect from carrying out a Juice Blitz and then following the High Life Diet? What is it going to do for you? What are the real payoffs?

The Bottom Line

There are many rewards to be gleaned from the Juice High lifestyle. Your body gets healthier, energy soars, skin is clearer and less wrinkled, eyes are brighter, weight problems lessen and chronic depression or anxiety start to become things of the past. But after all is said and done, the truth is that when it comes to regular juicing and a Raw Energy lifestyle, nothing less than *freedom* is the bottom line. Incorporating the power of Raw Energy day after day into your life not only brings freedom *from* negative experiences such as chronic fatigue and illness by strengthening immunity and deep cleansing of the body—it can also bring you freedom *to:* to be more creative and live out what you really are. The deep cleansing this kind of lifestyle brings and the regeneration that comes in its wake help set people free to live simply and joyously in the midst of all of the pollution, noise and conflict that surround them. For we live in a difficult time—a time which demands focused awareness and knowledge to handle not only the physical toxicity in our environment but also the spiritual and emotional toxicity that creates distortions in our perceptions and limits to the full expression of the unique soul energy which is embodied within each one of us.

If it surprises you that something as simple as following a way of eating and living that leaves out convenience foods—and is high in fresh raw produce and full of juicing—can affect how you see the world and how creative you can be in your life, then it is time to move beyond theory and test it all out by getting into your own juicing program. Then you can experience for yourself just how wonderful a personal revolution it can bring about. Detoxifying the body is a major step in finding and freeing the spirit. It can help you come to a way of living in which you are centered, clear and joyous the way a child is joyous—awakening in the morning with a sense of excitement about what the day ahead holds.

Expand Your Horizons

When you detox your body you remove impediments to experience and to action. You release energy that has been suppressed beneath the physical burden of waste that we all carry. But the thing about releasing energy is that the energy that is released needs to be channeled. For most people, the increase in energy that comes with a Juice High lifestyle grows gradually and steadily. Yet for some, it can be experienced as an explosion of life force that suddenly arises from within as if from nowhere. This was Leslie's experience the first time she ever did a juice fast. Working with a doctor who was an expert in detoxification, she began the experiment at his suggestion because she had an important decision to make about her life and she felt that she neither had the clarity nor the information she needed to be able to make it wisely. Her doctor friend has suggested that she try a fast. In the beginning this sounded completely insane to her. What possible bearing could drinking juices and water have on her decision making? Then he told her about all the ancient practices of using fasting for intellectual and spiritual ends. She learned how monks and nuns fasted to clarify their inner vision and bring them spiritual awareness, how Pythagoras fasted for 40 days and then insisted that his students fast also before sitting exams, and that the famous Swiss physician Paracelsus insisted that "of all the remedies available, fasting is the greatest one." And she began to wonder.

Gateway to Power

The Juice Blitz is but a milder form of detoxification than a fast on spring water. It will do the same thing but more slowly and more gently. And it is much easier on your system. It also has the advantage of not depleting your body of minerals and trace elements, as well as vitamins and other as yet unidentified metabolites that are central to high-level health. The High Life Diet will continue the detoxification processes—yet more slowly and more gently still—while it carries through the metabolic building process to help restore first-rate biochemical functioning on which high level health, emotional balance and mental and spiritual clarity depend.

So, Leslie—still unconvinced—began her juice fast, which she continued for 21 days under medical supervision. (This is the only way in which such a long juice fast should be carried out. More than two or three days on juice alone needs careful monitoring by a professional who understands and has experience with detoxification.) The results of her juicing quite literally changed her life. As a child she had suffered endless illness—colds, flu, high fevers and nightmares every night—while she was growing up. Then in her early twenties she had found herself imprisoned by a heavy long-term depression with no apparent cause for which no professional—doctor, psychologist or counselor, could find a cure. Unknown to her, it was juicing that would hold the key.

In the first five days on juice, she experienced the odd headache and a great deal of fatigue since her body was throwing off waste at a fantastic rate. This temporarily depleted her of energy for action so she rested. Then the whole world began to look different. Her body felt light instead of the burden she had for years experienced it to be. Her eyes grew bright. But what amazed her most of all was that her whole experience of who she was began to shift. So did the way she viewed herself, her life and the world around her.

SO EASY

Before her juice fast, she had experienced herself as someone struggling against great odds day by day to just to raise her children and find her place in the world. During the detox, she began to experience an ease about these things that she would never before have dreamed was possible. She noticed that her image of herself and her attitudes toward life were undergoing subtle yet profound shifts. Instead of experiencing herself as someone with a lot of limitations, confused about what she wanted to do and feeling that she could probably never do what she wanted to do even if she knew clearly what that was, she began to view herself as a simple, clear woman who with steady commitment and patience could accomplish what she wanted with her children and her work. She found that each day she would awaken without being riddled with anxiety as she had been before, and she would feel clear and excited about the day ahead.

Now, more than 20 years later, when Leslie thinks back to the revolution that took place in her own life as a result of juice fasting, she recalls a little story someone once told her, of a psychologist studying the nature of optimism and pessimism in children. It is a tale that perhaps describes better than her own words the changes that took place all those years ago—and she smiles. Here is the story:

In an attempt to understand the nature and functioning of the two personality types in children—the *optimist* and the *pessimist*—a group of psychologists set up an experiment. They took a large room and filled it with every conceivable kind of toy to amuse an eight-year-old—trains and trucks, building materials, stuffed toys, storybooks, painting and drawing materials. Then they took the eight-year-old *pessimist* and put him in the room while they and the child's mother waited in an adjoining office to see how long the child would amuse himself. In less than 10 minutes the child came out of the room whining, "Mommy, I am bored. There is nothing to do in there."

Next, the psychologists took the same room, removed everything from it replacing the toys, the books and all the rest with a large pile of horse manure. This time they sent an eight-year-old *optimist* into the room and closed the door then stood talking in the adjoining office expecting any moment for the child to come through the door. But he did not come. Instead, silence. Ten minutes passed. Then 20. Finally an hour went by with no sign of the child. After another 15 minutes, the child's mother voiced concern that perhaps her son had hurt himself. Deciding to indulge her concern, the psychologists let her open the door to see if her son were all right. Hearing the door open, the boy jumped up immediately and ran to his mother's arms shouting, "Mommy, Mommy, there's a pony in here but I can't find him."

Such is the power of detoxification.

Set Your Body Free

When it comes to physical strength and athletic prowess, juicing has real clout. After the Juice Blitz and ten days on the High Life Diet, your body becomes so much cleaner and clearer from inside out you no longer easily build up the wastes in the muscles and around joints that make exercisers and athletes so prone to injury. Also, since juicing and eating a diet high in raw fruits and vegetables tends to alkalinize the system, they are superb antidotes to the kind of acidic buildup that comes with exercise by which lactic acid interferes with being able to go on and on. Now you can work out longer and harder without pain. Replacing convenience foods full of junk fats, refined carbohydrates and chemical additives with fresh foods and live juices also gradually stabilizes blood sugar so that energy for physical activity is readily available and long lasting. After three months of juicing, one marathon runner described it this way: "Everything has become effortless. I can run longer and harder without straining. Instead of demanding so much of my will, I find myself almost floating over the hills and rocks. Just occasionally it gets so good, I feel as though I could run on forever."

Fuel For Change

We believe that the benefits of Juice High have the potential to be felt far beyond the individual. Social change is brought about by the dreams, the visions, the thoughts and the actions of people. The greater the clarity of perception and an individual's sense of freedom, the more creativity and potential benefit he or she can bring to work, relationships and society as a whole. Our educational system—despite the high-sounding phrases bandied around by politicians—is dedicated not to turning out free thinking, autonomous human beings but rather to "normalizing" thought and behavior. That way the status quo is maintained and potent, active eccentrics whose visions go against the grain are kept in close check.

The goal of Juice High is diametrically opposite to this way of thinking. It is about helping the individual strip away toxicity—whether intellectual, spiritual, physical or emotional—in order that he or she can stand tall with a clear mind and a clean body. As such it is a tool for helping to establish freedom of action at grass roots level—freedom for the person to act according to his or her perceptions and values and to pursue his or her own goals. And these are goals which arise from the core of one's being rather than those which have been imposed from outside by our parenting, our schooling or the exploitative ends of our materialistic society. Living the Juice High can help someone become genuinely free.

Freedom is not, as the advertisers would have us believe, drinking white rum on a tropical beach or wearing a pair of Levi 501s. Freedom is about living out the truth of your soul in the way you relate to others, in the work you do, in the creative pursuits and the choices you make. Of course, such freedom is profoundly dangerous to those structures which would control us by delivering a pastiche of the real thing. Yet such freedom is the greatest high any of us ever experience—far better than any drug could offer. It is the freedom of learning to trust yourself and living out the fullness of your being.

Future Change

Experiencing the kind of personal transformation that detoxification and metabolic body building bring helps individuals gain access to their own powerful individual visions and strengths. It can help them not to fit into a society which is itself ailing, but rather to change it in very practical, real ways so that gradually the world we live in can better support human life and the ecology of the planet. What is fascinating about real freedom is that it not only helps the individual experience and live out his own creativity and joy better, it also brings the very best that each of us has to offer to our families, communities and to the planet as a whole. And while it is certainly true that drinking a glass of green juice each morning and munching more carrots at lunch are not going to turn you into a Martin Luther King, Jr. or a Mother Teresa, it can go a long way toward helping you to clear away some of the physical, emotional and intellectual junk we have all picked up along the way that prevent us from being who we are, from seeing clearly and from trusting what we see and then acting on it. That is why we see Juice High as a practical, easy-to-use tool for personal transformation that can potentially lead toward social transformation of the deepest order. It is an exciting prospect.

RECIPES

There are several variables to be considered when formulating juice recipes. Fruit and vegetables have not yet been standardized (thank God) and vary considerably in size and juice yield. Not all centrifugal extractors are as efficient as others. Rather than give measurements in ounces, we decided that the most practical way to present these recipes is by indicating roughly how many pieces of fruit and vegetables you'll need to make approximately 280 milliliters/10 fluid ounces/half a pint.

Alfalfa—Father of All Juices

The word alfalfa means "father of all grains," and when it comes to hair health, you can't do better than alfalfa sprouts and carrot juice.

4–5 carrots
1 cup alfalfa sprouts
chopped parsley (optional)

Juice as usual and top with some chopped parsley and drink.

Apple & Pear

Apples and pears are closely related and make a sublime combination when juiced together.

2 pears
2 whole apples

Juice as usual and drink right away as this one oxidizes very quickly.

Apple, Celery & Fennel

2–3 apples
2 stalks celery
1 bulb of fennel

Apple, Pear & Berries

Berries are intensely flavored vitamin bombs that tend to be high in potassium and contain a remarkable range of other trace elements. Strawberries, raspberries, blackberries... in fact, any berry works well when blended with apple juice, or apple and pear.

2 apples
1 pear
12 berries (or as many as you like)

Reserve a couple of pieces of apple to put through the juicer last and to flush the thick berry juice through the machine.

Apple Zinger

A terrific breakfast-time enlivener that perks up the whole system and really wakes up your taste buds.

2–3 whole apples
1 whole lemon, peeled

1 or more 1/2-inch cubes of fresh ginger root

Juice as usual and serve.

Atomic Lift-Off

This is an excellent immediate lift when you are feeling low. It's also a wonderful chaser for shots of tequila!

4–6 ripe tomatoes

1 lime

pinch of cayenne pepper, or dash of Tabasco

Juice the tomatoes and the lime (removing the skin but leaving the pith) then sprinkle with a dash of cayenne pepper.

Beet, Carrot & Orange

Beet enriches the blood and provides an excellent tonic for the kidneys. The sweetness of orange juice in this recipe will help you become accustomed to the earthy flavor of beet.

1 smallish beet

1 orange

4 carrots

Save one of the carrots to put through the juicer last, as it will help to clear the machine.

Beet Treat

Profoundly powerful, this juice will give you sustained energy throughout the day.

1 beet (plus tops, if possible)

4 carrots

1 apple

1 stalk celery
1¼-inch section cucumber

Black Watermelon

You have two choices on how to prepare this: you can juice the skin of the watermelon as well as the pink flesh and then stir in the molasses. Or, you can take only the pink flesh, put it into a blender or food processor, add the molasses and blend. We prefer the second method, but both are good.

¼ small watermelon
1 tsp–1 tbsp blackstrap molasses (unsulphured)

Carrot & Apple

This is the most basic juice cocktail; use it as the springboard for experimentation. Start by combining equal parts of the two juices and experiment until you find the proportions that suit you; we prefer one part apple to two parts carrot.

4 carrots
1 apple

Carrot & Orange

1 orange
4 carrots

Peel the rind from oranges, but leave the pith, and put the whole fruit through the juicer together with the carrots.

Carrot Milk

Adding soymilk to freshly extracted carrot juice enhances its natural creaminess and gives you plenty of protein without the clogging effect of cow's milk. Try adding the juice of a single small parsnip —scrubbed, topped and tailed but not peeled—and a little grated nutmeg.

3 carrots
1 parsnip (optional)
soymilk to taste (or to fill the glass)
pinch of nutmeg

Carrot, Beet, Celery & Tomato

3 carrots
1/2 a beet, peeled
2 stalks celery
2 tomatoes

Carrot High

5 carrots
4 sticks celery
1 clove garlic

Juice as usual.

Celery Sticks

3–4 sticks celery
4–5 carrots
1 clove garlic

Juice as usual and drink immediately.

Chlorophyll Plus

handful dandelion leaves
handful parsley
handful spinach
1 whole apple
small bunch grapes

Citrusucculent

1 ripe grapefruit (or pink grapefruit)
1/2 of one ripe lemon
2 ripe oranges

Peel the fruit (leave the pith) and juice as usual.

Citrus Zinger

1 pink grapefruit
1 orange
1 apple
1/2 a lemon
1/2 a lime
1 or more 1/2-inch cubes of fresh ginger root (optional)

Cool as a Cuke

1 cucumber
1 clove garlic
1 tomato
dash of dill

Juice the vegetables and then sprinkle with ground dill
and serve over ice.

Cranberry Cocktail

1 cup cranberries
1 cup sweet grapes or 2–3 apples

Put the cranberries and grapes or apples through the juicer then add a squeeze of fresh lemon juice before serving. If you don't have fresh cranberries, you can use frozen ones.

Dandelion Plus

4–5 carrots
handful dandelion leaves
1 bulb fennel

Juice as usual, then squeeze a tablespoon of lemon juice to the mixture.

Double Whammy

4–5 carrots
handful dandelion leaves
2 whole pears

Easy Does It

1 whole large green apple
2 stalks celery
8–10 lettuce leaves

Juice as usual and drink before bedtime or when you are feeling particularly tense.

Fab 5 Fruit Juice

A great fruit punch, this recipe can be varied and different fruit substituted according to seasonal availability.

1/2 an apple
1/2 a pear
1 tangerine, or similar
12 grapes
1 peach

Fatty Acid Frolic

2 whole apples
2–3 dandelion leaves or large leaves of kale or beet tops
1 heaping tablespoon *fresh* vacuum-packed flaxseeds
1 very ripe banana

Juice the apple and leaves as usual. Put into a blender with the flaxseed and the banana and blend at high speed until smooth. Drink immediately.

Gingeroo

Carrot and apple juice tastes even better if you ginger it up a little:

1 or more 1/2-inch cubes of fresh ginger root
1 whole apple
4 carrots

Juice as usual, saving a carrot to put last through the juicer.

Ginger Berry

1 or more 1/2-inch cubes of fresh ginger root
1 medium bunch of grapes
2 cups blackberries or raspberries

Juice as usual. You can also add some sparkling mineral water to this or some ice; it makes a delicious and refreshing long drink on a hot day.

Ginger Spice

3 large carrots
1 whole pear
A small chunk of fresh root ginger

Put into the juicer and drink immediately.

Ginger's Best

1/2 cantaloupe

1/4-inch slice fresh ginger root

1 lime (peel, leaving pith)

Juice as usual.

Glorious Grapefruit

Apparently there is a world glut of pink grapefruit, which make a frothy sweet and sharp juice that we love to drink for breakfast. Peel the fruit, but remember to leave as much of the white pith as possible to put through your juicer. Two grapefruit will yield slightly more than half a pint of juice.

Green Friend

3 whole apples

2–3 dandelion leaves or a couple of large leaves of kale
   or beet tops

handful mint

Green Goddess

2 ounces carrot juice

2 ounces apple juice

2 ounces beet juice

2 ounces broccoli juice

1 tsp kelp powder

1 tsp chopped fresh parsley

squeeze fresh lemon juice

Green Satin

This is a delicious aromatic introduction to drinking green juices. Smooth as satin and beautiful to sip at sunset.

2–3 apples
2 stalks celery
bulb of fennel

Juice as usual.

Green Tomato

This invigorating green drink is not made with green tomatoes, which tend to be sour, but luscious red tomatoes.

2–3 ripe tomatoes
2 stalks celery
1 green pepper
1/2 bulb fennel
2–3 sprigs parsley/chopped parsley

Green Wild

2 green whole apples
2 stalks celery
1/4 lemon
1 or more 1/2-inch cubes of fresh ginger root

Juice together as usual, leaving the pith on the lemon, and serve.

Green Wow

2 green apples
4 stalks of celery
6 bok choy leaves
juice of half a cucumber

Green Zinger

2 leaves kale or beet tops or a handful of spinach
4–5 carrots
small handful parsley

Hi Mag

4–5 carrots
2 broccoli florets
2 leaves dandelion, beet tops, spinach or kale

Juice and season with a twist of lemon and a pinch
of salt.

Hi NRG

1 apple
2 carrots
1 stalk celery
soymilk to taste

Hit the Grass

handful fresh mint
small pineapple, peeled and cut into convenient-sized spears
handful of any fresh cereal grass such as wheat or barley

Juice the mint and pineapple in your ordinary juicer,
then juice the cereal grass in a wheatgrass juicer or,
alternatively, pour the fruit juice into a food processor
or blender and toss the cereal grasses in, blend with
the blade until highly blended, then pour through a
strainer to remove the indigestible fiber. Serve over ice.
This can also be made using a teaspoon to a tablespoon
of any of the freeze-dried cereal grasses such as barley
grass or wheatgrass.

Lazy Lettuce

2 whole apples
5 lettuce leaves

Lemon Zinger

1 whole apple
1/2 a lemon
Sparkling mineral water

Juice the apple and the lemon—leaving the white pith
on the lemon—pour into a glass and top up with
sparkling water and ice.

Leslie's Cocktail

*Bananas are not totally unjuiceable if you use very ripe
fruit. Put them through your juicer first, then juice the
apples, which will help to flush the thick banana through
the machine. Alternatively, use a blender to make the
breakfast of champions. This recipe also works well with
melon in place of apple.*

6 oz. fresh apple juice
1 ripe banana
1 teaspoon each spirulina, chlorella and green barley powder

Linusit Perfect

*This recipe is replete with valuable essential fatty acids—
both Omega 6 and Omega 3—which are often deficient
in people who have been surviving on the typical Western
fare of convenience foods. It must be made with vacuum-
packed flaxseeds or flaxseeds that are ground in
preparation, for these precious fatty acids are highly
unstable and go rancid quickly.*

2 whole apples
3 carrots
1/4-inch slice fresh ginger root
1 tablespoon flaxseeds

Juice the vegetable and fruit and ginger as usual. Place
the flaxseeds in a coffee grinder and chop up finely. Then
add to the glass of juice, stir well and drink immediately.
Alternatively, you can add the flaxseed to a food
processor, chop and then pour the freshly made juice in
and blend for three seconds.

Merry Belon

*Berries are one kind of fruit that combines really well with
melons and the array of flavors gives lots of scope for
experimentation. Try Galia & Raspberry, Honeydew &
Blackberry or the classic Watermelon & Strawberry.*

1 slice watermelon, 3 cm wide and cut into chunks to fit your
  juicer
6 strawberries, washed and with their green stalks removed

In hot weather, a good tip is to freeze your berries before
juicing them.

More Raw NRG

*When making this juice, put the ingredients through your
juicer in reverse order and you'll end up with a greenish
drink tinged with orange froth.*

3 carrots
1 apple
2 stalks celery
3-cm section cucumber
1 broccoli floret
small bunch spinach or watercress or dandelion leaves

Orange Tonic

2 oranges (remove the peel but not the pith)
1 or more 1/2-inch cubes of fresh ginger root
sparkling water

Juice the ginger and orange as usual, pour into a glass and top up with sparkling mineral water. This is particularly delicious in winter.

Parsley Passion

Another vegetable rich in mineral salts in parsley. Drinking parsley juice daily has brought relief to a number of people troubled by allergies.

1 bunch parsley
3–5 carrots
2 apples
2 small cauliflower florets

Papaya & Pineapple

This exotic combination is especially good for settling upset stomachs.

1/2 a small pineapple, cut into spears
1 mango

Take care to remove all the flesh from the stone of the mango before you juice it.

Parsnip Perfect

Parsnips, also known as anemic carrots, are well known for their ability to strengthen hair, skin and nails and can protect against hair loss.

2 parsnips
3 carrots
1 beet

Pepper Upper

This juice is a great replacement for coffee breaks and mid-afternoon pick-me-ups of caffeinated drinks and cookies. It helps you to sizzle with vitality without any of the downside you get from sugar and caffeine.

2 carrots
1 red pepper
1 stick celery
1/4 bunch of watercress
2–3 sprigs parsley

Save one of the carrots until last to clear out any juice left inside your machine. Otherwise, put the ingredients through in any order, stir and serve.

Pineamint/Pineapple Special

Especially good if taken at bedtime for settling the stomach and helping you sleep.

1 small pineapple
small bunch fresh mint leaves

Remove the skin of the pineapple and cut into convenient spears. Juice as usual. Serve over ice for a tall summer drink.

Pineappage

This may seem like a weird combination, but it's one way to sweeten the meganutrient fix of fresh cabbage.

1/4 large pineapple cut into spears
1/3 green cabbage

Juice as usual and drink right away.

Pineapple Grapefruit Drink

1 small pineapple
1 peeled grapefruit (peel but leave the white pith rich in
  bioflavonoids on)

Pineapple Green

6 oz. freshly pressed pineapple juice
1 tsp–1 tbsp of powdered wheatgrass, green barley, spirulina
  or chlorella

Popeye Punch

1 whole apple (including seeds)
4–5 carrots
small handful spinach
1 cucumber

Potassium Power

1 yellow or green melon, such as cantaloupe, honeydew, etc.
1 overripe banana
pinch grated nutmeg
6 cubes ice (made with spring water)

Scoop out the flesh of the melon, place in a food
processor or blender, add the banana, blend well and
pour into a glass over the ice cubes and sprinkle with a
pinch of freshly ground nutmeg.

Potassium Punch

*Our tribute to N. W. Walker, the raw food pioneer and
evangelist of detoxification; drink it religiously!*

3 carrots
2 stalks celery

4–6 leaves of lettuce or winter greens
handful spinach or watercress (or dandelion leaves)
few stalks fresh cilantro or parsley

Quantum Green

A super-charged blender drink enriched with sprouted pulses and sunflower seeds. Apples can be substituted for the pineapple.

3 carrots
2 spears pineapple
1/4 cup soaked sunflower seeds
1/4 cup assorted sprouts
handful spinach leaves.

Juice the spinach with the carrots, then cut the pineapple into chunks and put into the blender with the sprouts and seeds. Blend together, adding the freshly made juice.

Raw NRG

Carrot and apple juice is the basis for this health-packed cocktail, which is devised to promote all-around health with the addition of celery and cucumber, which both have a diuretic action that promotes elimination, helping your body to detoxify itself. As you become more adventurous in your juicing, try reducing the apple content and adding green leaves of cabbage, spinach or dandelion to increase the green energy content. Instead of using cucumber juice, you can top up with soy milk to create a creamy new Juice High experience. The addition of a cube or two of ginger gives the Raw NRG mix a real zing.

1 apple
4 carrots
1–2 stalks celery
5 cm section cucumber
1 or more 1/2-inch cubes of fresh ginger root (optional)

Red Cool

1 beet
2 apples
4 carrots
1 or more 1/2-inch cubes of fresh ginger root

Red Devil

This recipe provides a real tonic for the blood and is a great source of vitamins A, B-complex, C, D, beta carotene and vitamins K and E, as well as calcium, iron, potassium, magnesium, manganese, sulphur, iodine and copper. It's also useful for clearing infections of the urinary tract and upset stomachs.

3 carrots
3 stalks celery
1 beet

Put the carrots and celery in the juicer first and then add the beet. If feeling extravagant, serve with half a teaspoon of fresh cream floated on the top.

Red Flag

3 small ripe tomatoes
4 carrots
handful spinach

Red Genius

4 carrots

1 large raw beet

3-cm section cucumber

Rhubarb Radiance

2 large stalks rhubarb

3 medium apples

Juice as usual. Drink at night before bed.

Root Soup

Root vegetables are the best source of B-complex vitamins. Here, their thick, sweet and creamy juices are complemented by the anise-seed flavor of fennel. Dilute your root soup with cucumber juice, but if it's still too thick add a splash of spring water.

1/2 a smallish beet

1 medium-sized parsnip

1 sweet potato

1/2 a bulb of fennel

5-cm section cucumber

Salad Juice

4–5 carrots

4 sticks celery

3–4 radishes

Salsa Surprise

2 large ripe tomatoes

3 carrots

2 sticks celery

small bunch parsley
1 clove garlic

Secret of the Sea

2 whole apples
4 carrots
2 sheets nori seaweed

Juice the apple and carrot then pour into a blender
along with the seaweed. Blend thoroughly and serve.
This is even better if you toast the seaweed under a grill
or near a flame or hot plate very briefly—it takes no
more than 10 or 15 seconds to toast on both sides. You
can then break it up into the juice and blend.

Silky Strawberries

*Strawberries are surprisingly potent when it comes to
supporting a body that is under stress. Even one cup of
strawberries contains as much as 80 mg vitamin C,
minerals, plus all the other vitamins except for B12 and D.
Strawberries have a natural diuretic action and are very
calming to the liver. They also contain salicylic acid, which,
according to experts in natural medicine, is good for any
sort of kidney or joint complaint.*

2 cups strawberries
1 ripe pear
1 ripe banana
handful fresh mint leaves

Juice the strawberries and pear as usual then place in a
blender with the banana and mint and blend until
smooth. This drink is particularly delicious when made
with a frozen banana, it takes on the taste and
consistency of a natural ice cream.

Smooth as Silk

This recipe is rich in natural fruit sugars, potassium, magnesium and the amino acid tryptophan, which can be turned into serotonin in the brain. It is also absolutely irresistible.

2 cups blackberries, fresh or frozen
1 whole apple
1 ripe banana

Juice the berries and the apple. Put the juice and banana into a food processor or blender and blend until smooth. Drink 45 minutes before bedtime.

Spicy Apple

2 whole apples
1 lime
pinch cinnamon

Juice the apples and the lime (leave the pith on the lime), sprinkle with cinnamon and serve.

Spicy Carrot

This juice is a great source of minerals such as magnesium, potassium, calcium, iron, sulphur, copper, phosphorus and iodine, as well as antioxidants beta carotene, vitamins A, C, E and niacin, and vitamins D and K. It will also soothe a slightly delicate stomach.
Pineapples vary in size. You'll need half a small one or a quarter of a big one. Remove the fibrous skin with a sharp knife and cut into long spears that will fit into your juicer. Braeburn and Pippins are ideal for this juice, but any sweet apple will do.

4 carrots
2 spears of pineapple

1 Braeburn or Pippin apple
pinch ground cinnamon
pinch ground nutmeg

The cinnamon and nutmeg can be sprinkled on top of the freshly extracted juice or stirred into it, as you prefer.

Spiked Celery

4 stalks celery
4–5 carrots
1 clove garlic

Spinapple

When you mix apple with spinach, you have an amazing combination for cleansing the digestive tract and improving elimination quickly, probably because spinach, which is high in oxalic acid, combines with the pectin in mineral salts to form a unique compound that appears to have remarkable cleansing actions. Some practitioners in natural medicine claim that it actually clears old encrusted feces that has accumulated over months and years in the colon making it possible to eliminate it from the body.

3 whole apples
handful spinach

Juice as usual and drink twice a day, especially important just before bed.

Spring Salad

3 broccoli florets
4 carrots
2 stalks celery

1 clove garlic

1 tomato

Sprouting o' the Green

2 cups alfalfa sprouts

2 cups mung bean sprouts

1 carrot

a few sprigs parsley

2 apples

Sprout Special

This juice is rich in natural phytohormones that help protect the body from the damage that petrochemically derived pesticides and herbicides can foster. It is also enormously rich in life-enhancing enzymes.

4 carrots

1 whole apple

1 cup sprouted seeds (mung beans, alfalfa, chickpeas, adzuki beans, etc.)

Juice together as usual. You can sprinkle some grated ginger on top or a little cinnamon and serve over ice.

Straight CJ

When buying carrots, choose those with the darkest color. Size doesn't matter, but many of the recipes in this book refer to "medium-sized" carrots, around 6 inches in length. Whichever variety you use, you'll need about a pound of carrots to make 10 fluid ounces. As a rule of thumb, we reckon that half a dozen medium carrots will yield about half a pint of juice. Scrub them under cold running water and remove the tops and tails, but it is not necessary to peel carrots before putting them through the juicer.

Sweet & Spicy

2 apples whole
2 x 1/2-inch cube fresh ginger root
1/2 small pineapple cut into convenient-sized spears

Juice as usual, adding as much ginger as you like, and sprinkle with a little ground cinnamon.

Sweet Salvation

Bell peppers contain more vitamin C than oranges. Here, the juice is blended with freshly made tomato juice to produce a deep red-orange, sweet-savory drink.

1 red or yellow pepper
2 ripe tomatoes (or 1 beef tomato)
1 or 2 carrots
3 cm section of cucumber

Tomato & Carrot, Celery & Lime

A deliciously light combination (and not a bad medium for pepper vodka).

2–3 ripe tomatoes
2 carrots
2 stalks of celery
1/2 a lime

Top of the Beet

1 apple
5 carrots
3 leaves of beet tops
handful parsley

Tossled Carrot

5 big carrots
1 whole apple
pinch turmeric

Juice carrot and apple, pour into glasses and sprinkle
with turmeric.

Tropical Prune

1 small pineapple, peeled and cut into convenient-sized spears
2 fresh plums—when plums are not in season substitute
   one pear

Juice as normal, then grate a pinch of nutmeg on to the
top and serve.

Vegetaranian

4 carrots
1/2 bulb of fennel
1 apple
1 lime
handful fresh cereal grass or 1 tsp–1 tbsp powdered green
   supplements

Juice all ingredients except for the cereal grasses, then
put the juice and the cereal grasses in a blender or food
processor and blend thoroughly. Strain before serving to
remove the indigestible fiber. If you use a powdered
green supplement as well, then juice as normal, pour
the juice into the food processor or blender, add the
powdered green supplement, blend and serve over ice.

Virgin Mary

A Bloody Mary without the vodka, we find that the flavor of this refreshing tomato-based cocktail benefits from a few drops of Tabasco. Add a clove of garlic and it becomes a Vampire Mary; a fresh jalapeno or other hot green chili pepper turns it into a Scary Mary.

2 ripe tomatoes
2 carrots
1/2 a beet
1 stalk celery
1 cucumber

Waterfall

2-inch section cucumber
1 whole apple
3 carrots
1/2 a smallish beet

RESOURCES

Ingredients

Green Foods   Spirulina, chlorella, wheatgrass and green magma (the dried juice of young barley leaves) are available in various forms at Whole Foods locations nationwide, as well as many other health food stores. And be sure to check your local listings for farmers' markets.

Herbs   Bulk herb suppliers provide the most cost-efficient way to add tinctures, fluid extracts and loose dried herbs to your juices.

On the West Coast, try the Monterey Bay Spice Company, 719 Swift Street, Suite 62, Santa Cruz, CA 95060, telephone (800) 500-6148, www.herbco.com.

Based out of Iowa, the Frontier Natural Products Co-op is a leading provider of organic bulk herbs and spices to health food stores and apothecaries nationwide. Visit www.frontiercoop.com.

Honey   Visit the National Honey Board's database at www.honeylocator.com to find a honey producer and distributor that meets your needs.

On the East Coast, the Bee Flower & Sun Honey Co. specializes in local, raw honey, which they distribute nationally. Visit www.beeflowersunhoney.com.

On the West Coast, the Bear Foot Honey Farm has three generations of experience in beekeeping and honey production. Visit www.bearfoothoney.com.

Juicers   See EQUIPMENT.

Flaxseeds   Look for vacuum-packed varieties. Grind the seeds in a coffee grinder and sprinkle on cereals, salads, in yogurt or in drinks. Or put dry into a blender, grind them and pour on your fresh juice. Both whole seeds and flaxseed oil are available at Whole Foods and many other health food stores.

Vegetable Bouillon Powder   Seek out broth powder based on vegetables and sea salt and free from preservatives, available from health food stores. Low-salt forms are excellent for making spirulina broth.

Organic Foods   Seek out local farmers' markets, and check www.localharvest.org for lists of CSAs and organic farms in your area.

Sea Plants   Kelp, dulse, nori and kombu can be bought from Japanese grocers or macrobiotic health stores.

Soymilk   There are a number of good brands of unsweetened soymilk—a popular favorite is Silk, which can be found at most health food stores.

Equipment

The Juice Kitchen   Undoubtedly the most useful tool in the juice kitchen is a vegetable peeler. Not a blunt old potato peeler, but a speed peeler with a pivoting head which can be bought from any catering supply store if you can't find one in the local hardware store. Not all vegetables should be peeled, however, as their nutrients tend to be concentrated in the skin. Organic carrots, beets and apples are great juiced whole. Buy a scrubbing brush, such as a nail brush, to scrub the dirt off root vegetables. The brush will also be useful for scrubbing the strainer basket of your juicer.

Second, you need a sharp knife and a cutting board. If your chosen juicer has a spout rather than an integral jug, find some glasses that fit snugly under the spout, but buy an accurate measuring jug as well and use it to formulate your own recipes. Juicing directly into the glass saves on washing up, but it's useful to have a swizzle stick—a chopstick will do—or a thin wooden spoon to stir your juices before serving.

Domestic Centrifugal Extractors   Centrifugal juice extractors contain a basket, usually made from stainless steel, with sharp shredding blades at the bottom and a fine mesh screen at the sides. When you push fruit and vegetables through the rotating blades, the pulp is spun off into a receptacle at the back of the machine and the juice strained out through a spout, or into an integral jug. A juicer with a spout is better than one with a jug because then you can juice directly into a glass and there's less to wash.

As with any domestic appliance, when buying a centrifugal juicer, look for the most robust model you can get for your money. This means the one with the strongest motor and the strongest locking mechanism. Beware of two-speed juicers and those models with a hopper that simply clicks into place without you having to clamp it down. These rinky-dink features just give you more to go wrong.

One other thing to check before buying your juicer is the size of the hole you are supposed to put the produce through. Some are really too small and it's a drag to have to slice even the skinniest carrot lengthways.

Russell once took a burned out juicer back to the shop when it was less than a year old and the salesman asked how much he had used it. Actually, he'd used it every day, but what was it designed for? Don't be afraid to demand a demonstration of the model you intend to buy, listen to the whine the motor makes and ask yourself if it sounds like it can stand up to the job.

The Champion Masticating Juicer   Veteran juicers wax lyrical about the virtues of the Champion, an indestructible juicer that some people claim makes better juice than any centrifugal extractor can because its masticating action is more effective at "trituration," the process of splitting open the fibers of the plant matter and liberating its nutrients in the form of juice. The Champion is basically a rotating cutter on a shaft, which expels dry pulp from its shout at one end as the juice is drained through a nozzle underneath.

Expensive, the Champion is guaranteed for five years and can well last a lifetime, easily repaying the investment in the long run. For details of your nearest retailer, or to buy a Champion by mail order, contact the distributor: Quality Health Products Inc, 922 Black Diamond Way, Lodi, CA, 95240.

The Vita-Mix Total Nutrition Center   Basically a turbo-charged, super-efficient blender with indestructible stainless steel blades and an extremely powerful motor, the TNC is dynamite! It's the only machine that is properly able to make the fiber-rich juices—the kind of molecular, or total, juicing discussed in Chapter Nine. It is also effective for making cereal grass juices (which should be strained before drinking to remove indigestible cellulose fibers). The TNC not only makes juice, but can also be used to make soups and ice cream. The Super TNC can even be used to mix whole-grain bread. These machines are expensive, but owning one could change your life. Contact Vita-Mix for the name of a local distributor: Vita-Mix Corporation, 8615 Usher Road, Cleveland, OH 44138, telephone (216) 235-4840.

Sprouting

All you need to start your own indoor germinating "factory" are a few old jars, some pure water, fresh seeds/grains/legumes, and an area of your kitchen or a windowsill which is not absolutely freezing.

HOMEMADE SPROUTERS

There are two main ways to sprout seeds—in jars and in seed trays. Let's look at the traditional way first, then at the way we find easiest and best.

A simple and cheap sprouter can be anything from a bucket to a polythene bag. The traditional sprouter is a wide-mouthed glass jar. Some people like to make it all neat by covering the jar with a cheesecloth or a nylon or wire mesh and securing it with a rubber band, or using a mason jar with a screw-on rim to keep the cheesecloth in place. But we find the easiest and least fussy way is simply to use open jars and to cover a row of them with a tea towel to prevent dust and insects from getting in.

Start Here
- Put the seed/grain/legume of your choice, for example mung beans, in a large sieve. (For amount to use see the chart on page 205 and remember that most sprouts give a volume about eight times that of the dry seeds/grains/legumes.) Remove any

small stones, broken seeds or loose husks and rinse your sprouts well.

- Put the seeds in a jar and cover with a few inches of pure water. Rinsing can be done in tap water, but the initial soak, where the seeds absorb a lot of water to set their enzymes in action, is best done in spring, filtered or boiled and then cooled water, as the chlorine in tap water can inhibit germination—and is also not very good for you.

- Leave your sprouts to soak overnight, or as long as is needed.

- Pour off the soaking water—if none remains then you still have thirsty beans on your hands, so give them more water to absorb. The soaking water is good for watering houseplants. Some people like to use it in soups or drink it straight, but I find it extremely bitter. Also, the soaking water from some beans and grains contains phytates—nature's insecticides, which protect the vulnerable seeds in the soil from invasion by microorganisms. These phytates interfere with certain biological functions in man, including the absorption of many minerals (including zinc, magnesium and calcium), and are therefore best avoided. The soaking water from wheat, however, known as "rejuvelac," makes a wonderful liquid for preparing fermented cheese and is very good for you.

- Rinse the seeds either by pouring water through the cheesecloth top, swilling it around and pouring it off several times, or by tipping the seeds of the open-topped jars into a large sieve and rinsing them well under the tap before replacing them in the jar. Be sure that they are well drained either way, as too

Variety	Soak Time	Dry Measure	Days to Harvest	Sprouting Tips
Alfalfa	Overnight	3 tbsp	4–5	Grow on wet paper towel—place in light for last 24 hrs
Chickpea	Up to 24 hours	2c	3–4	Needs long soak; renew water twice during soak
Fenugreek	Overnight	1/2c	3–5	Pungent flavor
Lentil	Overnight	1c	3–5	Earthy flavor
Mung	Overnight	3/4c	3–5	Grow in the dark—place in light for last 24 hours

much water may cause them to rot. The cheesecloth-covered jars can be left tilted in a dish drainer to allow all the water to run out. Repeat this morning and night for most sprouts. During a very hot spell they may need a midday rinse, too.

- Return sprouter to a reasonably warm place. This can be under the sink or just in a corner not too far from a radiator. Sprouts grow fastest and best without light and in a temperature of about 70 degrees Fahrenheit.

- After about three to five days, your sprouts will be ready for a dose of chlorophyll if you want to give them one. Alfalfa thrive on a little sunlight after they've grown for two or three days, but mung beans, fenugreek and lentils are best off without it. Place them in the sunshine—a sunny windowsill is ideal—and watch them develop little green leaves. Be sure that they are kept moist and that they don't get too hot and roast!

- After a few hours in the sun, most sprouts are ready to be eaten. Optimum vitamin content occurs 50 to 96 hours after germination begins. They should be rinsed and eaten right away or stored in the refrigerator in an airtight container or sealed polythene bag. Some people dislike the taste of seed hulls such as those that come with mung sprouts. To remove them simply place the sprouts in a bowl and cover with water. Stir the sprouts gently. The seed hulls will float to the top and can be skimmed off with your hand.

NOTE FROM LESLIE

Make It Big   Now for my favorite and simplified method using seed trays. I find that, with the great demand of my family for living foods, the jar method simply doesn't produce enough. Also, for sprouted seeds, you have to rinse twice a day while tray sprouts need only a splash of water each day. This is a very simple way to grow even very large quantities easily.

Take a few small seed trays (the kind gardeners use to grow seedlings, with fine holes in the bottom for drainage). When germinating very tiny seeds such as alfalfa you will need to line your seed tray with damp, plain white kitchen towels. For larger seeds, the trays themselves are enough. Place the trays in a larger tray to catch the water that drains from them. Soak the seeds/grains/legumes overnight as in the jar method, then rinse them well and spread them a few layers deep in each of the trays. Spray the seeds with water (by putting them under the tap or by using a spray bottle) and leave in a warm place. Check the seeds each day and spray them again if they seem dry. If the seeds get too wet they will rot, so be careful not to overwater them. Larger seeds such as chick-peas, lentils and mung beans need to be gently turned over with your hand once a day to ensure that the seeds underneath are not suffocated. Alfalfa seeds can be simply sprinkled on damp paper towels and left alone and after four or five days will have grown into a thick green carpet. Don't forget to put the sprouts in some sunlight for a day or so to develop lots of chlorophyll. When the seeds are ready, harvest them, rinse them well in a sieve and put them in an airtight container or sealed polythene bag until you want them. To make the next batch, rinse the trays well and begin again.

TIPS AND TRICKS

Some sprouts are more difficult to grow than others, but usually if seeds fail to germinate at all it is because they are too old and no longer viable. It is always worth buying top-quality seeds because, after removing dead and broken seeds and taking germinating failures into account, they work out to be a better value than cheaper ones. Also try to avoid seeds treated with insecticide or fungicide mixtures such as those which are sold in gardening shops and some nurseries. Health food stores and large grocery stores are usually your best bet, as is anywhere you can buy seeds very cheaply for sprouting in bulk. It is fun to experiment with growing all kinds of sprouts from radish seeds to soybeans, but avoid plants whose greens are known to be poisonous, such as the deadly nightshade family, potato and tomato seeds. Also avoid kidney beans, which are poisonous raw.

Some of the easiest to begin with are alfalfa seeds, adzuki beans, mung beans, lentils, fenugreek seeds, radish seeds, chickpeas and wheat. Others include sunflower seeds, pumpkin seeds, sesame seeds, buckwheat, flax, mint, red clover and triticale. These latter can sometimes be difficult to find or to sprout—the "seeds" must be in their hulls and the nuts must be really fresh and undamaged. Good luck!

SPROUTING CEREAL GRASSES

You will need:
> seed-tray (or a kitchen tray will do)
> good organic potting compost
> 8–10 layers of newspaper
> sheet of plastic to cover the tray
> seed—hard red winter wheat or buckwheat, barley etc.

How to sprout:

1. Soak approximately 1 cup seeds for 12 hours in water to cover well, pour off the water and allow to drain for 12 hours.
2. Half-fill the seed-tray with compost (so that the compost comes halfway up the sides of the tray), level the surface and spray with a fine spray of water. Make sure you do not soak the compost.
3. Place the soaked seeds on the wet soil so that the seeds are evenly spread and not on top of each other.
4. Soak the newspaper thoroughly, cut to the size of the seed tray and cover the seeds. Place the plastic on top of the newspaper.
5. Leave the tray in a well-ventilated, not overwarm room for three days.
6. At the end of three days, remove the plastic and newspaper and put the trays somewhere where they will get plenty of light—a sunny window sill for instance—and water once a day, making sure you do not soak the soil.

7. In about five to eight days the plants should be six-
   to eight-inches high and standing tall and green.
   They are then ready to cut.
8. Cut the greens close to the soil with a sharp knife.
   They can be kept in the fridge in plastic bags for
   several days.

Cereal grasses can be grown all year-round wherever
you live and regardless of whether you have a garden. Use
organic seed, which should be available from good health
food stores. Cereal grasses can only be juiced using a
machine specifically designed for this purpose.

Alternatively they can be put into a powerful blender,
such as the Vita-Mix, with ½ a cup of raw fresh juice or
spring water and blended for 10 to 20 seconds to pulverize
them. Then you need to strain away the indigestible cellulose before serving.

FURTHER READING

Good Diet

The Bircher Benner Health Guide. Ruth Kunz-Bircher. London: Unwin Paperbacks, 1981.

Diet and Salad Suggestions. Norwalk Press, Arizona: N. W. Walker, 1940.

Dr. Bircher-Benner's Way to Positive Health and Vitality 1867-1967. Zurich: Verlag Bircher-Benner Erlenback-1967.

Eating Your Way to Health. Ruth Bircher Benner. London: Faber and Faber, 1961.

Life in the Twentieth Century. Richard Taska Jr. Woodstock Valley, CT: Omangod Press,1981.

Macrobiotic Diet. Michio & Aveline Kushi. Tokyo and New York: Japan Publications, 1993.

Nutrition Against Disease. R. Williams. New York: Pitman Publishing Co., 1971.

Nutrition and Physical Degeneration. Weston A. Price. La Mesa, CA: Price-Pottenger Nutritional Foundation, 1970.

Nutrition for Vegetarians. Agatha Moody Thrash, MD & Calvin L. Thrash, MD. Seale, AL: Thrash Publications, 1982.

The Prevention of Incurable Disease. M. Bircher-Benner. Cambridge: James Clarke & Co., 1981.

Subtle Energies in Foods

A Cancer Therapy. Max Gerson. Del Mar, CA: Totality Books, 1977.

Dr. Bircher-Benner's Way to Positive Health and Vitality 1867-1967. Zurich: Verlag Bircher-Benner Erlenbach, 1967.

The Electromagnetic Energy in Foods. Dr. Hazel Parcells. Albuquerque, New Mexico: Par-X-Cell School of Scientific Nutrition, 1974.

The Essene Science of Life. E. B. Szekely. Cartago, Costa Rica: International Biogenic Society, 1978.

Food Science for All. M. O. Bircher-Benner. London: C.W. Daniel, 1928.

Man and Biologically Active Substances. I. I. Brekhman. Oxford: Pergamon Press, 1980.

The Phenomena of Life: A Radio-Electrical Interpretation. George Crile. New York: W. W. Norton, 1936.

The Prevention of Incurable Disease. M. Bircher-Benner. Cambridge: James Clarke & Co., 1981.

What Is Life? and Mind and Matter? Erwin Schrodinger. Cambridge: Cambridge University Press, 1980.

Green Foods and Drinks

Cereal Grass. Ed., Ronald L. Seibold, MS. New Canaan, CT: Keats Publishing Inc., 1991.

Chlorella. Dr. David Steenblock. El Toro, CA: Aging Research Institute, 1987.

The Magic of Green Buckwheat. Kate Spencer. Romany Herb Products Limited, 1987.

Nature's Healing Grasses. H. E. Kirchner. Riverside, CA: H. C. White Publications, date unknown.

Real Health Starts With Eating Light. Mitsuo Koda MD. Privately published.

The Wheatgrass Book. Ann Wigmore. Wayne, NJ: Avery Publishing Group Inc., 1985.

Wheatgrass Juice. Betsey Russell Manning. Calistoga, CA: Greensward Press, 1994.

Why George Should Eat Broccoli. Paul A. Stitt. Milwaukee, Wisconsin: The Dougherty Company, 1990.

Wild Foods

Wild Food. Roger Phillips. London: Orbis Publishing, 1983.

Rejuvenation

Become Younger. N. W. Walker, D.Sc. Phoenix, AZ: Norwalk Press, 1949.

The New Ageless Aging. Leslie Kenton. London: Vermilion, 1995.

Therapeutic Use of Juice and Foods

Encyclopaedia of Healing Juices. John Heinerman. New York: Parker Publishing Company, 1994.

Food Power. George Schwartz, MD. New York: McGraw-Hill Book Company, 1979.

Total Juicing. Elaine LaLanne with Richard Beyno. Plume, 1992.

Food Enzymes & Health

Enzymes & Enzyme Therapy. Anthony J. Cichoke, DC. New Canaan, CT: Keats Publishing Inc., 1994.

Enzyme Nutrition. Dr. Edward Howell. Wayne, NJ: Avery Publishing Group Inc., 1985.

Enzymes The Foundation of Life. D. A. Lopez, MD; R. M. Williams, MD, PhD & M. Miehlke, MD. Charleston, SC: The Neville Press Inc., 1994.

Energetic Nutrition

A Cancer Therapy. Max Gerson. Del Mar, CA: Totality Books, 1977.

"A Turning Point in Nutritional Science." R. Bircher. *Lee Foundation for Nutritional Research*, no. 80.

Dr. Bircher-Benner's Way to Positive Health and Vitality 1867-1967. Zurich: Verlag Bircher-Benner Erlenback, 1967.

The Essene Science of Life. E. B. Szekely. Cartago, Costa Rica: International Biogenic Society, 1978.

Food Science for All. M. O. Bircher-Benner. London: C. W. Daniel, 1928.

Man and Biologically Active Substances. I. I. Brekhman. Oxford: Pergamon Press, 1980.

The New Raw Energy. Leslie & Susannah Kenton. London: Ebury Press, Vermillion Press, 1994.

The Phenomena of Life: A Radio-Electrical Interpretaion. George Crile. New York: W. W. Norton, 1936.

The Prevention of Incurable Disease. M. Bircher-Benner. Cambridge: James Clarke & Co, 1981.

What Is Life? and Mind and Matter? Erwin Schrodinger. Cambridge: Cambridge University Press, 1980.

Juices & Juicing

Raw Vegetable Juices. N. Walker. New York: Jove Publications Inc., 1977.

INDEX

ABOUT THE AUTHOR

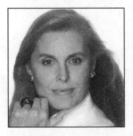 **Leslie Kenton**, an award-winning writer, television broadcaster and teacher, is well-known for her no-nonsense approach. Highly respected for her in-depth reporting, she is described as "the most original voice in health and beauty" and the "guru of health and fitness." A consultant to the European Parliament for the Green Party and course developer for Britain's Open University, Leslie is responsible for more than 40 bestselling books on health, beauty and spirituality, including one novel and a memoir. Trained in acupuncture, nutrition, bioenergetics, and energy medicine, she is a member of AAMET and NTCB in the U.S. and a certified homeotheraputics consultant. Leslie lectures and teaches natural methods of enhancing health, creativity and personal power which enable people to gain more control over their own lives and make better use of their personal creativity. You can find out more about her at www.lesliekenton.com and www.curaromana.com.